Premature
Babies

Sherri Nance (signature)

by Sherri Nance

With Sharon Timmons

and Marilyn Bick, Leslie Kane, Tina Kauffman, Kay

Nash, Sherry Pearson, Patty Turney, Darleena Wade and

Joanne Williams

Darleena Wade (signature)

Kay Nash (signature)

Premature
Babies
A HANDBOOK
FOR PARENTS

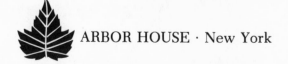

ARBOR HOUSE · New York

To the children . . .

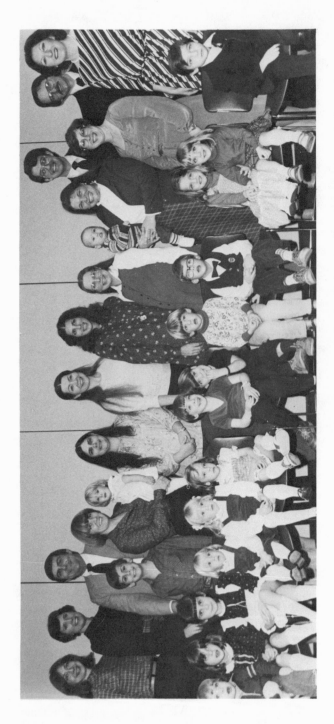

PREMATURE, INC. MEMBERS AND THEIR FAMILIES Front row: (seated, left to right) Matthew Kahn, Jennifer Kahn, Karen Turney, Suzanne Bick, Johanna Bick, Mindy Wade, Zachary Pearson, Jeffrey Pearson, Tyson Kane, Michael Williams, Monica Nance, Susan Timmons, and Trey Nash. Back row: (standing, left to right) Susan Kahn, Patty Turney, Bill Turney with Bobby Turney, Marilyn Bick holding Elizabeth Bick, Darleena Wade, Sherry Pearson, Leslie Kane, Joanne Williams, Sherri Nance holding Jonathan Nance, Patrick F. Timmons, Jr., Sharon Timmons, George Nash and Kay Nash. *Credit: Craig Stotts*

Contents

8

Preface

In 1976, by divine providence or fate, five mothers who had delivered their children prematurely and a perinatal social worker, all of whom were interested in concepts of parent support, found each other.

These six women and several of their husbands were the first members of the Parents of Prematures in Houston, Texas, organized under the Houston Organization for Parent Education, Inc. (HOPE). They began as an informal group, meeting in members' homes over coffee, tea and formula to share the common problems they had in parenting premature infants. The group grew quickly, and members found that no matter what their individual experiences had been, they shared common feelings. They had all felt the frustration of leaving tiny newborns in hospital nurseries in a society where most mothers carry home round-faced term babies in their arms.

As quickly as these parents realized their own needs, the purposes of the group expanded and were altered. They formed a telephone support committee and started a hospital visitation program. To do so, they developed contacts and a rapport within the local medical community. They also assumed the responsibility of becoming a paraprofessional volunteer organization. A steering committee was established to plan projects and oversee activities. HOPE was petitioned for monetary support. Dreams became long-term goals.

Parents of Prematures was in the right place at the right time.

The mailing list blossomed into several pages. Members were asked to speak at neonatal staff meetings in major hospitals, perinatal workshops, a statewide perinatal conference, local high school classes. A videotape of an interview with a panel of members was filmed for social workers and nurses in Houston who would deal with parents of premature infants. Two mothers designed patterns for premie clothing, and successfully arranged for a manufacturer to market one of the first commercially sold lines of premature infant garments available in the United States. A survey of over 100 parents was undertaken. "Premie packets" were created for distribution.

And a thought that had been floating through several minds for two years finally took shape: There has got to be a book written on the experiences of parents of premature infants. No such book existed. True to the logic used in accomplishing other projects, group members asked, "Why can't we write the book?"

A core assembly of approximately a dozen people saw the project from beginning to completion. They decided what the book should be—a support book for married couples who have had premature infants. They brainstormed the initial outline, wrote of their own experiences, solicited other parents to write, dissected the intermediate drafts. When publication seemed imminent, they became a separate, nonprofit organization, Premature, Inc., to deal with the legal and financial obligations and liabilities of working as a group.

.... And all this while, continuing with their own lives. Several held full-time jobs. A number had subsequent pregnancies, ending both prematurely and at term. Some suffered major tragedies. A few moved away from Houston but stayed active.

The activities of the support group as a whole continued. Book meetings were held, with children crawling onto other parents' laps, spitting up on notebooks, eating chapter pages, racing through living rooms.... And then there were months when the group met twice a week, and fathers stayed home with children so that mothers could argue in peace and quiet. . . .

This group accomplished what many thought would be impossible: They were friends, who worked on a professional task for three years with no personal remuneration—for two years the group worked with almost no money at all—and they remained friends. This book, whose royalties will go to the organization, was an act of love and in some ways a labor of gratefulness—for financial assistance during hard times, for the emotional support of others, for children who survived and were basically healthy. They worked because they knew the book was needed.

After notices were placed in national parenting magazines about the writing of the book, replies were received from across the United States that not only confirmed the group's convictions, but also served as their reward. A mother from Florida wrote:

> Throughout the past two years I've vowed more than once that I should write a book on prematurity or at least share my thoughts on paper with other mothers who have had premature infants. This lack of information regarding this subject is phenomenal.

And a parent from Chicago:

> Congratulations on your fine undertaking. I only wish there had been a book like yours eight years ago. Since there wasn't, I look forward to reading it now.

And from Houston:

> I felt so fortunate to have had my low-birth-weight baby in Houston, and one of the reasons is because of the tremendous support I received from your group.
>
> It was such a great help to be able to talk to someone with similar experiences at a time when I really needed to know that others had survived such an ordeal . . . .
>
> Your book fills such a great need. I applaud each of your members for their hard work and extraordinary efforts!

In writing this book, the group researched the statistics regarding premature birth. We learned that 300,000 premies are born annually in the United States. We found that 75 percent of these infants grow up without any serious medical problems.

More than statistics, however, parents need support. Parents of premature infants find strength in knowing that someone else has a small, ill baby who was left in a hospital, and that the parents of that baby emotionally survived.

Sherri Nance
Houston, Texas

Foreword

Premature birth is recognized as a world health problem. About 7 percent of liveborn infants are born weighing 5½ pounds or less. In the United States there are 250,000–300,000 low-birth-weight infants born each year. Neonatal mortality is about twenty times greater for these infants than for infants who weigh more than 5½ pounds at birth.

However, during the past two decades, dramatic changes have taken place in the approach to perinatal care and the management of the newborn infant. The successful survival of premature infants provided by intensive care has prompted special intensive care management of all high-risk newborns. Credit for rate of survival and decreased mortality among premature babies must be shared by obstetricians, pediatricians, nurses, laboratory and paramedical personnel. It is our greatest hope that every infant have the potential of a full productive life and life expectancy.

But while medical care is excellent, parents of prematures have lacked adequate emotional support. Recognition of this need has led to the development of the group, Parents of Prematures.

Parents of Prematures is a volunteer service organization of parents who have had a premature child. Its objective is to provide support to other parents of prematures through personal visitations in the hospital and home, telephone communications, and dissemination of information on prematurity. Parents of

13

Prematures, founded in 1976, was the first group of its kind in Houston and has continued to be one of the most active groups in the country, having since spawned other groups nationally. The phenomenal success of the group results from several factors: (1) The core group composed of sensitive, assertive, intelligent people interested in giving support to other parents; (2) The high value placed on shared information among parents and professionals; (3) The support and backing of the medical community in Houston.

This book reflects all three. Drawing on their own experience as well as their contacts with hundreds of other parents of prematures, the authors have gathered together crucial information to guide parents through all the problems, fears, hopes, confusion and concern engendered by premature birth. Carefully researched and scientifically accurate, the latest medical and nursing information is carefully explained in easy to understand terms, as are the practical aspects of feeding, dressing and caring for a premature baby. A complete, practical handbook, the physical and psychological needs of both parents and babies are discussed in detail.

Parents of Prematures initially perceived the need for a book on premature birth at the local level, but as they became involved, they realized the need for this vital information to be made available nationally.

Since no book of this kind currently exists, and because it is the single item most requested by new parents of prematures in their initial contact with Parents of Prematures, this publication will undoubtedly be invaluable in dealing with the very special problems of premature babies.

I trust that it will have a vigorous life and long and honorable existence.

Arnold J. Rudolph, M.D.
Professor of Pediatrics, Obstetrics & Gynecology
Director, Newborn Section
Baylor College of Medicine
Houston, Texas

Acknowledgments

Compiling a book like this is a monumental task. Literally hundreds of people made contributions of one sort or another in order to see the dream of a book specifically for parents of premature infants become a reality.

Members of Premature, Inc., took responsibility for compiling information and stories, writing, editing and preparing the manuscript for publication. The following twenty people freely donated their time and talents to this project: Barbie Beach, San Antonio, Texas; Marilyn Bick, Bellaire, Texas; Susan Bork, Westlake, Ohio; Jeanette Geron, Ballwin, Missouri; Ella Beth Goetschius, Houston, Texas; Susan Kahn, Bellaire, Texas; Leslie Kane, M.S.W., A.C.S.W., Houston, Texas; Tina Kauffman, Alamo, California; Cindy Mahon, Houston, Texas; Carolyn Meyer, Houston, Texas; Sherri Nance, Houston, Texas; Kay Nash, Houston, Texas; Sherry Pearson, Conroe, Texas; Terri Schenck, Clarinda, Iowa; Jill Thrift Schlansker, Ph.D., San Antonio, Texas; Patrick F. Timmons, Jr., Houston, Texas; Sharon Timmons, Houston, Texas; Patty Turney, Houston, Texas; Darleena Wade, Houston, Texas; Joanne Williams, Houston, Texas.

In addition to Premature, Inc., members, there were several parents and professionals who participated in early meetings of the Parents of Prematures Book Committee. Their opinions and suggestions helped shape the book. Thanks go to the following people who attended those first meetings: Nance Cohen, Houston, Texas; Emma Fox, R.N., Houston, Texas; Lee Ann Kelley,

R.N., Houston, Texas; Martha Ogburn, R.N., Greenville, North Carolina; and Charlene Quast, Missouri City, Texas.

While not every person who contributed to this project will find his or her words printed in the book, each one who responded to our call for personal stories provided ideas vital to making the book as complete as it is, and all of them confirmed the need for a book like this. To the following individuals and couples, we offer sincere thanks for their willingness to share their thoughts and experiences: Mary C. Anderson, Conroe, Texas; Kathleen G. Auerbach, Ph.D., Omaha, Nebraska; Kelley J. and Robert Barnes, Frederick, Colorado; Judith Bea, Boulder, Colorado; Barbie and Doug Beach, San Antonio, Texas; Patricia Beifuss, Painesville, Ohio; Marilyn and Harry Bick, Bellaire, Texas; Sally Blair, Houston, Texas; Terry Blakley, Fort Worth, Texas; Susan and Joe Bork, Westlake, Ohio; Mardell Bowie, Houston, Texas; Sherry Brandt, Spring, Texas; T. Berry Brazelton, M.D., Boston, Massachusetts; Peggy and James Breef, Houston, Texas; Peggy Brown, Scotch Plains, New Jersey; Pat D. and Scott Burton, Lakewood, Colorado; Cheryl Busbice, M.S.W., Houston, Texas; Janice Butler, Fort Walton Beach, Florida; Kaye W. Carter, Houston, Texas; Susan Clark, Pleasant Hill, California; Cindy Cleveland, Littleton, Colorado; Michelle Cockerille, Manassas, Virginia; Nance Cohen, Houston, Texas; Cathlyn Coon, Bellville, Texas; Jim Courtney, M.D., Houston, Texas; Lynda de los Santos, Houston, Texas; Debra DeSharnais, Santa Fe, New Mexico; Murdina M. Desmond, M.D., Houston, Texas; Pamela Dickerson, Noblesville, Indiana; Coral Dicks, R.N., Houston, Texas; Angela Dinwiddie, Houston, Texas; Marcia Driscoll, Walnut Creek, California; Monica A. Ficaretta, Bowie, Maryland; Kim Fischer, Albuquerque, New Mexico; Suzanne Fitzsimmons, Houston, Texas; Judi Ganem, Cape Neddick, Maine; Jeanette and Steve Geron, Ballwin, Missouri; Evangeline Godron, Moose Jaw, Saskatchewan, Canada; Ella Beth and David Goetschius, Houston, Texas; Janet Gonzalez-Mena, Suisun, California; Alice Gottschling, Norman, Oklahoma; Suzanne G. Green, Houston, Texas; Bobbie A. Henderson, Ph.D., Houston, Texas; Rose Herzog, R.N., Longview, Texas; Dianne Veillon Hill, Houston, Texas; Reba Michels Hill, M.D., Houston, Texas; Meredith Holly, Houston, Texas; Cindy Hood, Eugene, Oregon; Debbie

Acknowledgments 17

Jackson, R.N., Houston, Texas; Alvin Jaffee, M.D., Houston, Texas; L. L. James, M.D., Houston, Texas; Lauree D. Janak, Danville, California; Susan and Eddie Kahn, Bellaire, Texas; Virginia Kallus, Houston, Texas; Leslie Kane, M.S.W., A.C.S.W., Houston, Texas; Tina and Richard Kauffman, Alamo, California; Karen Kendrick, L.P.T., Houston, Texas; Carol Kennon, Houston, Texas; Sheldon Korones, M.D., Memphis, Tennessee; Marjorie Kuhn, Glidden, Texas; Carol and John Lacouture, Littleton, Colorado; Pamela and Jim Latham, Livermore, California; Lauri Lowen, Bellevue, Washington; Cindy and Larry Mahon, Houston, Texas; Nona H. Mason, Houston, Texas; Susan B. McCoy, R.N., Denver, Colorado; Linda R. and Jim McKee, Houston, Texas; Carolyn and Charles Meyer, Houston, Texas; Cynthia Moore, The Woodlands, Texas; Suzanne Nabona, Pearland, Texas; Sherri and Daryel Nance, Houston, Texas; Donna Nash, Houston, Texas; Gail Nash, Houston, Texas; Kay and George Nash, Houston, Texas; Martha Ogburn, R.N., Greenville, North Carolina; Libby Orlando, Houston, Texas; Debbie Parnell, Porter, Texas; Sherry and Chet Pearson, Conroe, Texas; Theresa and Charles Pope, Akron, Ohio; Wendy Powell, Kansas City, Missouri; Rosemary Price, El Paso, Texas; Julie A. Prince, Katy, Texas; Charlene Quast, Missouri City, Texas; Sally Ruth Rau, Chicago, Illinois; Bonnie Rowley, Sunset Hills, Missouri; Rebecca Werne Sanchez, Virginia Beach, Virginia; Rev. Robert Saxby, Wichita Falls, Texas; Teri Schenck, Clarinda, Iowa; Jill Thrift Schlansker, Ph.D., San Antonio, Texas; Reed Schmidt, San Francisco, California; Lois Scott, Linden, Colorado; Roberta Siegel, R.N., Denver, Colorado; Emily Selig, Denver, Colorado; Anita K. Shelangowski, Champaign, Illinois; Debbie Smith, Mendota Heights, Minnesota; Shirley Sobolewski, Forestville, Maryland; Joyce Stagg, Texarkana, Texas; Fran Stanford, M.D., Houston, Texas; Joan Stuhrenberg, Palacios, Texas; Cathy Sunkel, Hurst, Texas; Jennifer L. Sutton, R.N., Houston, Texas; Ron Taylor, Boulder, Colorado; Richard M. Thaller, M.D., Houston, Texas; Sharon W. and Patrick F. Timmons, Jr., Houston, Texas; Susan Tuohey, Houston, Texas; Patty and Bill Turney, Houston, Texas; Alan G. Van Orman, M.D., Cardston, Alberta, Canada; Kathy Vandenberg, Oakland, California; Barbara Vernier, Richmond, Texas; Darleena and Milton Wade, Houston, Texas; Lisa

Wagner, R.N., Houston, Texas; Linda Watson, Houston, Texas; Debra K. Wehrle, Houston, Texas; Nancy Weiner, Sharon, Massachusetts; Debbie L. Westheimer, Batavia, Ohio; Rulena White, R.N., Houston, Texas; Beth Williams, Gibsonia, Pennsylvania; Joanne and Bob Williams, Houston, Texas; Linda R. and Steven M. Wilmoth, The Woodlands, Texas; Sheryl and Ken Wilson, Antioch, California; Denise Winter, Fenton, Missouri; Cindy Zauss, El Cajon, California; Barbara Zeagler, R.N., Houston, Texas; Diane Abshire-Smith and Ron Smith, Fairfield, California; Annette Barker, Houston, Texas; Mildred M. Brady, L.V.N., Houston, Texas; Edna Coutts, R.N., Houston, Texas; C. Monroe Copeland, Houston, Texas; Mary S. Gregory, Houston, Texas; Mr. and Mrs. H. M. Grounds, Houston, Texas; Sharon D. Hermann, R.N, Houston, Texas; Phyllis Wilmoth, R.R.T., Houston, Texas; Geraldine McKnight, Suitland, Maryland; Paula and Ron McWherter, Houston, Texas; Paulette and Orlando E. Nelson, Houston, Texas; Shirley Northrup, Houston, Texas; Mary Ann and Thomas B. O'Donnell, Liberty, Texas; Lynda L. Panzica, Houston, Texas; Gwenn Pobanz, Spring, Texas; Prudence Podratz, Houston, Texas; Vasuki Ramakrishnan, M.D., Houston, Texas; Michael J. Rice, Houston, Texas; Helen Slape, R.N., Houston, Texas; Lucille Smith, R.N., Houston, Texas; Laura A. Whooley, R.N., Houston Texas.

Special mention must be made of the professionals in Houston, among them Dr. Arnold J. Rudolph, Dr. Reba Michels Hill, Dr. Murdina M. Desmond, Dr. Joseph A. Garcia-Prats, Dr. James Adams and Dr. Clark M. Hinkley. They encouraged and supported us, reviewed chapters for us and assisted in many other ways.

We also appreciate the March of Dimes National Foundation and Houston hospitals—Jefferson Davis Hospital, Hermann Hospital, St. Joseph's Hospital, Texas Children's Hospital, Woman's Hospital of Texas—and the Meyer Center for Developmental Pediatrics for their help in obtaining photographs. The following individuals deserve our thanks for their assistance: John Blecha, March of Dimes; Peggy Cleary, Martha Lyons, R.N.—and Barbara Merritt, R.N., Jefferson Davis Hospital; Edna Coutts, R.N., Hermann Hospital; Jane Pohodich, R.N., and Mary DeJong, R.N., St. Joseph's Hospital, and Mary Nesbitt, R.N., Woman's Hospital of Texas. Craig Stotts, R.N., also deserves much credit for his sensitive photographs.

Several manufacturers and companies were also helpful in providing information or photographs or both, among them, Lopuco, Gomco, Egnell, Happy Family Products, Tiny Mite Premie Fashions, Critikon and Vickers Medical Ltd.

And finally, there are a few people and organizations that contributed other skills, services and information: Mike Blumenfeld, Houston, Texas; Kaye Campbell, Houston, Texas; Alicia Conklin, New York, New York; Susan Daley, Westlake, Ohio; Lorelei de la Reza, Houston, Texas; Leroy J. Dierker, M.D., Cleveland, Ohio; Ellen Galinsky, Palisades, New York; Houston Organization for Parent Education, Houston, Texas; Carole Kennon, M.S.W., A.C.S.W., Washington, D.C.; Melinda Kwong, M.D., Buffalo, New York; La Leche League, International, Franklin Park, Illinois; Vicki Lansky, Deephaven, Minnesota; National Association of Perinatal Social Workers, Oklahoma City, Oklahoma; Mary Paez, Houston, Texas; Chet Pearson, Houston, Texas; Eddie Pevey, Heights Funeral Home, Houston, Texas; Ridgway's, Houston, Texas; Lois Schlehuber of Premie Clothing, Etc., Houston, Texas; and Bob Williams, Houston, Texas; Sherli Wislon, Houston Texas.

Chapter 1

PREMATURITY

On August 2, 1979, Chaya Snyder, whose first name means "life" in Hebrew, was born weighing 15 ounces. Delivered at twenty-six weeks gestational age, this first child of Robert and Fay Snyder was not quite 15½ inches long at birth. Chaya, whose weight dropped to 13 ounces in the days after birth, was developmentally normal at the age of one year.

Nine months before Chaya's birth, Mignon Faulkner was born weighing 17 ounces and measuring 12 inches in length. Mignon was delivered during her mother's twenty-third week of pregnancy, and she lived in San Diego Children's Hospital a year before she was released, when she weighed 10 pounds 9 ounces. She was on a respirator for seven months, and reports indicate that she may have a slight hearing loss. Mignon was the fourth premature infant born to her parents. During Mignon's hospital stay, a sign furnished by her mother was tacked above her incubator. It read, "Please be patient. God isn't finished with me yet."

These babies, among the smallest who have survived premature birth, are only two of thousands who are delivered too early each year.

When such babies make a sudden, unprepared entry into this world, parents likewise enter an unfamiliar territory. This "world" of neonatal units, specialized techniques of care, and technological marvels is at the leading edge of the medical frontier.

At first glimpse, a neonatal intensive care unit may seem to parents to be a place where the future has come to life. The foreign language of a relatively young medical field, neonatology, assaults their ears. Their minds may be filled with confusion and doubt. They often feel numb; they are in shock. Each conversation or report is like an unpredictable wind, whipping their emotions one way and then another, from feelings of joy to fear and then back again. Living with such emotional extremes is mentally and physically exhausting. Premature birth is a crisis for everyone involved—parents, professionals and babies.

No one intends to have a premature baby, but when birth does occur too early despite the best efforts of doctors, all must face the situation and deal with it. Often parents feel a heavy burden of loneliness as they attempt to cope with this threat to their parenthood. In truth, they are not alone. They are usually surrounded by caring professionals, relatives and friends. Other parents, too, have had the same feelings, the same thoughts. Similar problems have been faced before by others.

Members of the parent support group that compiled this book know from personal experience what questions are likely to be raised in parents' minds. These questions form the foundation of this first chapter, which offers basic information about prematurity in order to help parents better understand the facts they are given by the professionals who so skillfully care for their babies.

BORN TOO EARLY: WHAT IT MEANS

Parents first of all need to know the meanings of some medical terms. The glossary, beginning on page 000, provides simplified definitions.

To the medical community, a *premature* infant is one born prior to the completion of the thirty-seventh week of gestation and usually weighing less than 2,500 grams. This 1969 definition by the World Health Organization was a revision of a 1948 WHO statement in which prematurity was defined solely in terms of birth weight. Over the years, confusion arose because there are babies born at term who weigh less than 2,500 grams. In redefining prematurity, it was suggested the word *preterm* replace premature. However, at present most parents and the public are unfamiliar with this term and continue to use premature in describing a baby born too early.

To further simplify the definition, "premies," as such babies are affectionately known, are infants born two or more weeks early and generally weighing less than 5½ pounds. This does not mean that premies are simply small babies. The lungs, nervous system, stomach and other body organs and systems of these babies are not mature. This immaturity can cause temporary or permanent problems with breathing, heart action, control of temperature and blood sugar levels, jaundice and other complications. The natural immunities and stores of iron that are built up in a baby during the last few months of pregnancy are limited or nonexistent in premies. As a result, they are often susceptible to infection. Even if these small babies encounter no critical medical problems, they may have difficulty sucking, a reflex that develops in the last trimester of pregnancy, and may, therefore, have problems eating and gaining weight.

Many premies do not have eyelashes or fingernails. Cartilage may not have formed the shape of the ears. A boy may be born before his foreskin has grown or his testicles have descended. A girl may have a prominent clitoris and small vaginal folds. The child is sometimes covered with fine hair, called lanugo, that ordinarily is sloughed off in the womb.

These infants, who by all rights should not yet be born, are a paradox. Attempting to create artificial wombs is not the best way to care for them, because birth itself has triggered biological mechanisms necessary to life outside the womb. The preterm baby is "an organism in an environment he has not yet evolved for." (Tiffany Martini Field, ed, *Infants* Born at Risk: Behavior and Development)

Although incubators, respirators, tube feeding and other extraordinary means of keeping the children alive try to duplicate womblike conditions as much as possible and as far as needed, these babies are required at birth to accomplish the amazing feat of breathing room air, often with immature lungs.

Premature infants may occasionally "forget" to breathe. In some premies, these spells, called apnea, may occur rather frequently. An undetected episode of apnea can cause a slowed heart rate, called bradycardia, and lead to sudden death. Detected, an apnea spell can usually be halted by as little stimulus as jarring the infant's crib or thumping his foot. More serious or frequent apnea spells can require medication, ventilation or other forms of treatment.

Not all low-birth-weight infants are premature. Infants born either at term or prematurely and weighing less than 2,500 grams can also be classified as "small for date" or "small for gestational age" (SGA). SGA infants are physically small in terms of weight, but their systems are usually appropriately developed for their gestational age. In such cases, placental insufficiency, the mother's ill health, smoking, drinking, exposure to drugs, malnutrition or unknown causes may be responsible for the baby's small size.

Like SGA infants, "true" prematures, or those born before full prenatal development has occurred, generally have grown and developed appropriately for the length of time they have spent in utero. They are small because their period of uterine development has been cut short. Several studies have indicated that premies, unless brain damaged or otherwise handicapped, tend to "catch up" with infants born at term in most areas of development by their second year of life. A widely accepted but sometimes disputed theory among child-development specialists holds that until age two, a prematurely born child's development needs to be thought of in terms of an "adjusted age"—that is, calendar age minus the number of weeks the child was born early. (A six-month-old infant born three months, or twelve weeks, early would have an adjusted age of three months.) Even considering adjusted age, parents should realize that some premies need time to "put everything together" in terms of integrating and coordinating all of the body's complex systems. (Murdina M. Desmond, "Parenting the Premature Baby")

Developmental milestones often do not occur at the ages listed in popular child-development books. For example, some premies who do not crawl until their eleventh month proceed to crawl, sit up and walk before their first birthday. In a few areas, these infants have been rushed into maturity in their struggle to survive. The most obvious example is that they are required to breathe on their own and take food by mouth earlier than they would have if they had been delivered at term. In other areas, premies may develop more slowly than the norm for even their adjusted ages.

On the other hand, SGA infants are generally at a greater disadvantage in terms of future development and growth whether born at term or prematurely. However, even a majority of SGA infants grow up quite normally.

CAUSES OF PREMATURITY

A major concern of most parents is discovering the reason why their baby was born too soon. However, it is frequently impossible for doctors to pinpoint immediately a cause for the premature birth. It is estimated that 50 percent of all premature infants are delivered early for unknown reasons. The main known causes of prematurity are multiple births, toxemia, incompetent cervix, placenta previa, abruptio placentae, inadequate diet, and drug and alcohol abuse.

Multiple Births

The uterus is designed to carry one baby. The conception of twins, triplets or more can cause additional weight that the mother's body may be unable to carry to term. The additional strains on the mother's systems may prove too great to sustain the pregnancy. While multiple births are frequently a few weeks early, extremely early delivery may point to other possible causes.

Toxemia

Toxemia of pregnancy is a major cause of maternal and infant death. It consists of two phases: preeclampsia and eclampsia. The first phase is characterized by swelling, leaking of protein into the urine and elevated blood pressure, especially after the twenty-fourth week of pregnancy. In the second phase, a woman may have seizures and go into a coma. Delivery of the infant is the only cure for the second stage of toxemia. Even after delivery, the mother's life remains at risk. In such cases, delivery of a relatively healthy baby, even if prematurely, is considered a significant achievement.

Incompetent Cervix

Incompetent cervix is a condition in which the cervix is unable to remain closed until the pregnancy reaches term. Dilation and effacement usually occur during the second or early part of the third trimester due to a mechanical defect of the cervix. Incompetent cervix may be hereditary or the result of poor childhood diet or trauma (damage to the cervix that occurs during a previous delivery, dilatation and curettage [D and C] or abortion).

Exposure to DES (diethylstilbestrol) has also been linked to incompetent cervix, as well as to uterine abnormalities that may prevent a woman from carrying a baby to term. DES is a synthetic estrogen-type hormone that was prescribed by doctors in the 1940s and 1950s to prevent miscarriage. Recent research has indicated that the drug did not in fact prolong threatened pregnancies, but it did affect the babies whose mothers took the drug. Some DES daughters have been found to have an unusual type of vaginal or cervical cancer. More commonly, those exposed have noncancerous tissue changes or structural changes in the vagina or cervix.

Any woman who believes that her mother took DES while pregnant should consult her doctor about possible problems in future pregnancies. Additional information about DES and its effects are available at federally funded DES clinics located throughout the country and from the National Cancer Institute, Office of Cancer Communications, Bethesda, Maryland 20205.

Placenta Previa

The uterus is shaped like an inverted bottle. In placenta previa, the placenta implants itself in the lower part of the uterus, too close to the neck of the womb. A portion or all of the placenta blocks the cervix or birth canal. As the baby grows and the uterus expands, placental blood vessels break, resulting in a painless, bright red bleeding that can be severe or minimal, depending on the size of the blood vessels that are broken. The causes of placenta previa are generally unknown, but the condition can be detected by X ray or sonography. If the placenta migrates upward, a normal vaginal delivery can occur. In most cases, however, the placenta does not migrate and a Cesarean section must be performed for the safety of the child and the mother.

Abruptio Placentae

In abruptio placentae, the placenta becomes partly or entirely detached from the lining of the womb before the baby is born. If complete detachment occurs, the baby will die in utero. Partial separation can affect the baby's growth while in the womb. Generally a mother is unaware of this condition, but with good prenatal care, abruptio placentae can be diagnosed.

Insufficient Diet

In recent years, much attention has been given to the effects of nutrition upon the fetus. Studies of pregnant animals have shown that insufficient diet can indeed affect the developing baby. Statistics on prematurity are often correlated with economic status, and researchers have noted that mothers who live on the poverty level cannot or do not always eat well. As a result, many of their babies are born too early and too small. Other mothers with busy schedules may not eat properly.

The question of weight gain during pregnancy has generated some controversy recently, but most doctors and nutritionists do agree that pregnant women should eat balanced, nutritious meals, avoiding "junk" foods or overly refined foods. Following a weight-loss diet during pregnancy can have dire consequences for the baby that the mother is carrying.

Drug and Alcohol Abuse

An alcoholic mother has an alcoholic baby growing inside her. A mother who is addicted to drugs delivers a drug addict who goes through withdrawal symptoms after birth.

The effects of a mother's drinking and drug addiction can be disastrous for her baby. The infant is born with the possibility of having physical, mental and behavioral abnormalities that may be impossible to overcome.

Drug and alcohol abuse are more often thought of in connection with SGA infants, but they can also be a cause of prematurity. Some specialists feel that it might be the life-style of the user more than the drugs themselves that causes early birth. These mothers may not eat well. If they go through withdrawal during pregnancy, the shock to the system can bring on labor.

Diabetes

Diabetes is a health complication in the mother that can cause prematurity or indicate the need for elective premature delivery. Premature infants of diabetic mothers often weigh more than 2,500 grams. Despite their size, these infants, too, have immature body organs and systems.

Rh Negativity

In a case of Rh negativity, where the mother carries a child whose Rh factor is negative, the infant can develop the disease known as erythroblastosis fetalis. Today the incidence of this disease is less common, as pregnant women are screened for the possibility of Rh problems, and methods of handling the matter have been greatly improved. In some cases, however, a premature delivery may be elected by the doctors caring for the mother and her baby, especially if the environment of the womb is judged to be more hostile to the infant than life outside the womb.

Hydramnios

Hydramnios, which is also sometimes referred to as polyhydramnios, is the excessive accumulation of amniotic fluid. This condition is caused by known as well as unknown factors.

Miscellaneous Causes

Abnormalities of the uterus, infections of the amniotic fluid, accidents, and C-sections or induced vaginal deliveries performed too early as a result of miscalculation of the due date can lead to prematurity. Premature rupture of the membranes almost always results in premature delivery. Smoking and environmental factors, such as pollution, have also been linked to early births. A correlation between the incidence of repeated induced abortions and prematurity has been observed in this country and in several East European countries where abortion is a commonly used method of birth control. (Cynthia W. Cooke and Susan Dworkin, *The MS. Guide to a Woman's Health*)

Unknown Causes

The unknown reasons for having a premie can be more frightening to parents than known causes. The unknown hangs like a ghost in a forgotten closet over the conception and delivery of subsequent children.

An initial, overwhelming question for most mothers, and sometimes fathers, regarding the delivery of a premature infant is "Why?" They wonder, "Did I work too hard? Did I lift something too heavy? Did I try to do too much? Should we not have had intercourse recently? Why did this happen?"

Even when the cause of premature birth is unknown, a doctor may suggest a reason for the early delivery. One obstetrician told a mother that her membranes may have ruptured as a result of a sudden change in barometric pressure. One mother questioned the influence of microwave radiation. A couple in California was told that the husband's exposure to Agent Orange, a defoliant used in Vietnam, could have played a part in their child's prematurity and a previous miscarriage. Some mothers have had the feeling that their children were simply ready to be born.

So much is still unclear. More premies are born during particular seasons. No one knows for certain why this occurs. Even with the enormous strides made by medical research, doctors still do not know exactly what triggers labor.

EFFECTS OF PREMATURITY

A premature birth affects parents primarily on a psychological level, while the most obvious effects on the baby are physical. Researchers admit, however, that infants may also be affected psychologically. At present, information on such psychological effects is unavailable.

On the physical level, there are three areas in which the effects of prematurity are most pronounced: (1) weight and feeding, (2) temperature control and (3) susceptibility to disease and medical complications.

The weight loss commonly sustained by all infants after birth is more pronounced in premies, for whom the loss of a few ounces may be a substantial percentage of the total weight. Feeding the premature infant can be complicated by a number of factors, among them the lack of a sucking ability or rooting reflex, the amount of energy expended in sucking, a need for extra calories, the size of the infant's mouth in relation to the size of the mother's nipple, the development of a lactose intolerance or medical complications in the abdomen or intestines. Depending on the specific problems, doctors may use IVs, continuous nasogastric (N/G) tube feedings, gavage feedings or other means of providing the child with nourishment.

Almost all premature babies lack subcutaneous fat, the thermal layer directly under the skin that assists the child in temperature regulation. Control of body temperature is also influenced by the fact that the infant's nervous system is immature—the baby cannot shiver or sweat—and that the surface area of the baby's body is large in comparison to weight. Constant monitoring by a sensor attached to the infant's skin is used to insure that the infant is neither too cool nor too warm. In either case, the child uses extra calories in the effort to regulate body temperature.

Because of their immature organs and systems, premature infants are highly susceptible to disease and medical complications. Such complications include respiratory (breathing) difficulties, cardiovascular (heart) problems, hematologic (blood) imbalances, renal (kidney) complications, ophthalmic (eye) problems and a general lowered immunity to disease. This susceptibility makes the infants' first days and months of life critical. Many doctors feel that a premature baby's first seventy-two hours are the most critical, but parents should be aware that after that time setbacks and new problems can still occur.

One old wives' tale that parents are likely to hear or remember is that infants born at the end of the seventh month are more likely to survive than those born in the eighth month. This superstition comes from the ancient Greeks, who believed that a baby was responsible for its own birth. Greek physicians thought that the fetus literally kicked and wiggled its way into the world. They reasoned that if a fetus tried to "escape" from the uterus at the end of the seventh month and succeeded, it was strong. However, if it failed, another attempt at birth was repeated in the eighth month, and the fetus, now exhausted by its previous effort, was more likely to die. Since, in actuality, the infant's maturity is generally the key to survival, each day the baby remains in utero increases the odds for survival.

While prematurity is related to a number of serious medical and developmental problems, it is also important to realize that with the advent of improved medical technology and techniques, the outcome of prematurity has been vastly improved. Fewer premies die now, and more survive without significant or long-term disabilities or handicaps.

CARE OF PREMIES

The next questions on parents' minds are usually about the baby's care and how parents can help. Neonatal intensive care units (NICUs) and premature nurseries, with their specially trained professionals, can be threatening or reassuring.

Reactions to such care vary. The following response of a new mother is typical:

> I finally saw him two days after he was born. Even though my husband had told me how tiny Will was and what intensive care was like, I was not prepared for what I saw. Tiny babies, machines humming and blinking, alarms sounding, everything was noisy and bright.
>
> Will looked like a tiny bird. There was no fat on his body, and his bones were so small. I was surprised to see that he had hair, nails and eyebrows, but no rear end. His premature diaper was so big that he just lay on top of it.
>
> His tubes, bilirubin lights and monitors were hard for me to cope with. It all seemed so unreal. I was afraid to touch him for fear he'd break.
>
> His nurse talked to us about his condition. She was very factual, but I could sense how much she cared. I was having a hard time understanding what had happened. All I could do was cry and wonder, "Why did this have to happen to me?"

Another mother's reaction to the NICU where her daughter was cared for was a bit different:

> My fears for Bonni's first seventy-two hours of life were greatly magnified when I was told that she had been admitted to an intensive care unit . . . . Four days after her birth, I visited Bonni in Neo and discovered that my worst fears were unfounded.
>
> The unit was wallpapered in a juvenile print fit for a nursery. There were large windows on all sides of the room . . . . Best of all, I . . . found the doctors and nurses to be people dedicated to saving the lives of these tiny neonates.

In most of the hospitals where premies receive care, parents are welcomed into the nursery by a medical staff that understands the need of parents to visit and relate to this new member of their family. However, in a few hospitals, nursery doors remain closed, just as they did in earlier times.

In their book and articles on maternal-infant bonding, Dr. Marshall H. Klaus and Dr. John H. Kennell offer interesting insights into the changing attitudes regarding the care of hospitalized premature infants and the role of their parents. They point out that in the 1890s the French physician, Dr. Pierre C. Budin, one of the first doctors to be interested in the care of newborns, advocated maternal visitation for premies, breast-feeding and use of his glass-walled modification of the incubator so that mothers could see their infants more easily. In caring for these babies, Budin recognized the potential danger of separating a mother and her child. In his book, *The Nursling,* published in 1907, he wrote, "Unfortunately . . . a certain number of mothers abandon the babies whose needs they have not had to meet and in whom they have lost all interest. The life of the little one has been saved, it is true, but at the cost of the mother." (Pierre C. Budin, *The Nursling: The Feeding and Hygiene of Premature and Full-Term Infants*)

Budin, in seeking approval for his method of caring for premature infants, sent his student, Dr. Martin A. Couney, to the Berlin Exposition of 1896 to demonstrate that these infants could survive. German doctors, who did not believe that premature babies were viable, willingly allowed Couney to display them in his *kinderbrutanstalt,* or child hatchery. The display was a clinical and commercial success. Couney then exhibited tiny infants in incubators at fairs in England, where he was not so well received, and in the United States, settling on Coney Island.

Over a thirty-nine-year period, Couney cared for more than 5,000 premature infants. Although he followed most of Budin's precepts, he did make one notable exception: Mothers were not allowed to assist in the care of their own infants. They were merely given free passes to see the babies. Klaus and Kennell point to the revealing fact that Couney had difficulty persuading the mothers of some of these exhibition babies to take their infants home once they had attained a weight of 5 pounds. (Marshall H. Klaus and John H. Kennell, *Maternal-Infant Bonding*)

Despite the commercial aspects of Couney's handling of premature infants, many of his methods—and his attitude toward parents—were adopted by the first premature nurseries established in the United States. This exclusion of parents from active participation in caring for their hospitalized infants lasted until the late 1960s when changes in concepts of newborn care began to be promoted. Before that time, hospitals recommended only the most essential handling of the infants and a policy of strict isolation. Germs were enemies, and family members were carriers of germs. As late as 1970, a survey indicated that only one-third of the premature nurseries in the United States permitted parents into the nursery to visit their infants.[6]

PARENTS: THEIR EXPECTATIONS AND ROLES IN BABY'S CARE

Parents who are allowed into the nursery and are permitted to care for their baby in small ways find that the expectations they had during pregnancy about their child, infant care and a host of other related matters must be modified, and sometimes completely changed. Hospitalized premature infants do not act, and should not be expected to act, like full-term infants. These babies are simply not supposed to be born yet. Parents who are unfamiliar with premies often wonder, "Why do premies sleep all of the time? Why don't they cry? What exactly do they do?"

It is true that these babies sleep a great deal, just as they would if they had remained in utero. It is not true that these babies do not cry. Premies do cry, but their crying cannot be heard when they have tubes in their throats. Later when the tubes have been removed, their throats may be so sore that crying is too painful.

Basically what a premie does while in the hospital is struggle to survive, while continuing to develop and grow. The care that premies receive attempts to enable them to survive and develop in the best possible way. Parents are called upon to supplement

[6] Ibid., p. 116.

that care with the emotional support and love that only they can provide. An infant attached to four heart-monitor pads and wires, a temperature probe, an N/G tube and an IV usually can be wrapped in blankets and held. Eyes bandaged during photo-therapy for jaundice can be uncovered and therapy temporarily halted so that parents and infants can share in the intimacy of visual contact.

Premature infants need the presence and support of their parents, if at all possible, even if they can be together only for infrequent visits in a restricted setting. Parents, too, feel the need for contact with their infants despite the discomfort they may feel in this new and confusing hospital world.

Chapter 2

FINDING YOUR WAY AROUND THE HOSPITAL

"The hospital is difficult to adapt to. It brings in individuals from outside, and plunges them into a totally new existence, with new schedules, new food, new rules, new clothing, new language, new sounds and smells, fears and rewards. For the patient . . . there are no guides or guidebooks. . . . A person visiting Europe can get better advance information than a person entering the foreign country of the hospital." (Michael Crichton, *Five Patients: The Hospital Explained*)

ENTERING THE MAZE

Even the most well-planned hospital with direction signs clearly visible at the intersection of each set of halls can seem like a maze to newcomers. For parents of hospitalized premies, the maze extends to the numerous nursery units where their child will receive care. An infant who is improving or who has a setback may be moved from one nursery to another; infants' hospital "beds" are frequently rearranged to make the best use of space. When parents arrive for a visit, they often must "find" their infant all over again.

The infants are brought to the units in various ways—transferred from a home or hospital by ambulance, airplane or helicopter or taken to the nursery from a labor and delivery area in the same hospital. Most parents know little about the equipment, staff and policies that will so greatly affect their lives and their infants in the coming days, weeks or months.

They generally are also unfamiliar with the hospital services they will encounter or can request. Although each hospital is unique, there are services that are commonly available.

NURSERIES

In 1977, the Committee on Perinatal Health prepared a report, entitled *Toward Improving the Outcome of Pregnancy*. It recommended the systematic regionalization of perinatal care, *perinatal* referring to care of the pregnant woman before birth and care of the infant after birth. The committee outlined and classified three levels of care, offering suggested guidelines for each level. Although adoption of this terminology is not yet universal, a review of the committee's explanations can be helpful in understanding the equipment, staffing and procedures in nurseries.

Level I. These hospitals, with a low number of deliveries, primarily provide services for uncomplicated maternity and newborn patients. Emphasis is placed on earliest possible recognition of high-risk cases to facilitate consultation, referral and transport of the mother or infant to a Level II or Level III center.

Level II. Level II units exist in large urban and suburban hospitals where the majority of deliveries occur. These units provide a full range of services for uncomplicated perinatal cases, in addition to services for the majority of complicated obstetrical problems and certain neonatal illnesses. These units have a well-trained staff competent to deal with many but not all perinatal problems and up-to-date, well-maintained equipment needed to handle such problems. Level II units are not equipped to deal with the most serious, complicated cases and refer such cases to Level III units.

Level III. Level III units, often referred to as *regional perinatal centers,* are not only prepared to care for all normal and unusual perinatal cases, but they are charged to "provide leadership in preparatory and continuing education to improve the overall quality of care in the region and in generating, developing and evaluating new concepts and techniques in prenatal and perinatal care." (Committee on Perinatal Health, *Toward Improving the Outcome of Pregnancy: Recommendations for the Regional Development of Maternal and Perinatal Health Services*) Level III units are expected to be actively involved in perinatal research.

These three levels of care are translated into several different types of nurseries where premies are taken after birth, depending upon their medical condition. At community or small outlying hospitals, one area of the regular nursery is usually set aside for premature infants. Babies who are born prematurely at these hospitals and who have no medical complications stay at the hospital where they are born until ready for discharge. Some suburban hospitals or those in medium- to large-size cities have separate premature or intermediate care nurseries where help is available for babies who have serious, but not life-threatening, complications. Large urban hospitals or those in medical centers or regional perinatal centers usually have neonatal intensive care units, premature nurseries and one or two intermediate care nurseries.

UNITS FOR PREMIES

In a smaller hospital's nursery area for premies—a premature nursery and an intermediate care unit—parents can expect the following:

> • The baby will probably be in an incubator, since premature infants have difficulty maintaining their body temperature. A heat sensor (ISC probe), consisting of a pad

and wire, may be taped to the infant's body or attached with an adhesive.

- The infant's head may be shaved so that an IV can be placed in the scalp where veins are larger and more accessible.
- The baby may wear a heart monitor. If so, four small, spongy disks with wires connected to the monitor are attached by adhesive to the infant's chest and thighs.
- Since the infant cannot cough up mucus, a small plastic tube connected to a vacuum may be used to remove mucus from the nose, mouth or trachea.
- Most premies are initially fed by a tube that leads from the nose or mouth to the stomach. This method, called gavage feeding, is used because premature infants are often born before they have developed a sucking reflex or because doctors want to minimize weight loss by conserving calories that would otherwise be expended in trying to eat. If the capacity of the infant's stomach is extremely small, the nasogastric tube may be left in place so that the baby can be fed by a drip method. This continual feeding is monitored by machine.

Although vital to the baby's health, the seemingly endless number of wires and monitors can be disconcerting to parents. One mother writes:

A few hours later, he was off of any breathing machines, but he remained on a heart monitor, ISC probe and feeding tube. I was starting to wonder if I would know my son without tape across his cheeks and between his nose and mouth.

NEONATAL INTENSIVE CARE UNITS

In a neonatal intensive care unit, a medical team cares for sick infants. One nurse is usually available for every one or two infants, and physicians and therapists are on call twenty-four hours a day. The physician in charge of the unit is a neonatologist. In an NICU, the following is common:

- There will be some incubators, but most infants will be on warmers, which are tablelike beds warmed by lights from an overhead canopy and easily accessible to doctors and nurses.
- Large TV-screen monitors are often placed high upon the wall or attached to the ceiling. Each monitor is connected to the heart-monitor pads and wires on one infant. The monitor allows the medical staff to see at a glance the baby's heart rate, respiration rate and blood pressure. If the baby has an apnea spell, an alarm will sound.
- A baby with jaundice will be under bilirubin lights for phototherapy. An infant undergoing such treatment wears no clothes or diaper but does wear a protective eyepatch or blindfold. During phototherapy, a jaundiced baby's yellow skin may become suntanned. The baby's color eventually returns to normal.
- An infant who has great difficulty breathing or fails to breathe spontaneously may be placed on a respirator, a machine that assumes control of the baby's breathing by delivering oxygen to the lungs through an endotracheal tube (from the nose or mouth) at appropriate intervals. If an infant's lung collapses, called a pneumothorax, a chest tube, used to expand the lung, is inserted into the pleural cavity through a small opening made in the chest.
- Babies who require oxygen may be placed under a clear plastic hood attached to a hose. The oxygen is often humidified, making it difficult to see the baby's face through the foggy hood.
- The infant is likely to have a bandage on each heel, since blood for various tests, such as a complete blood count or bilirubin check, is obtained by pricking the infant's heels.

Parents may find it difficult to visit the NICU. It is a busy, noisy place where the atmosphere is often tense, reflecting the serious nature of what is happening there. To some parents, this maze of machines, wires and hoses is disturbing or overwhelming. Others quickly see past the technology and focus on their baby.

You've probably never seen an intensive care . . . nursery. You walk through the door and the first thing you feel is the intense heat. All around you are machines. Machines that beep, machines that have flashing lights, machines that are buzzing and counting. In the midst of some enormous monster called a warmer lies your baby . . . . There are wires and tubes everywhere. You think, "Is that my baby! It looks like a little old man." His skin is wrinkled. His hands and feet look enormous. Your baby looks different than the babies you have seen in the nursery, but he is your baby and you love him.

EQUIPMENT

For specific medical problems, an infant may temporarily need other specialized equipment or procedures. Since neonatology is a new and constantly changing field, what is used on one infant may not be used on another infant with the same problem in the same hospital a year later. The following are examples of such specialized equipment or procedures:

- A CAT (computerized axial tomography) scan may be used to detect or verify suspected internal problems. The CAT scan, actually a nuclear X-ray machine, provides computerized, three-dimensional X rays that show more detail than is possible on a conventional X ray.
- An infant screening audiometer is used in intensive care nurseries to identify infants who may have moderately severe to profound hearing loss.
- An electrocardiogram (EKG) may be ordered for the baby. The electrocardiograph records changes in heart action, and the resulting EKG tracing assists doctors in diagnosing heart problems or abnormalities.
- Doctors may use an electroencephalograph to detect and record the infant's brain waves. The electroencephalogram (EEG) shows the pattern of the brain waves; an abnormal pattern may indicate that the brain has been damaged.
- A heat shield is a small plastic dome that is placed over

an infant's body to decrease heat loss.

- A stomach pump is often used if the child requires abdominal or intestinal surgery.
- Doctors may use an umbilical artery catheter (UAC) on the baby. The UAC is a small plastic tube that is inserted into the artery in the infant's navel. In some instances, a radial artery catheter (RAC), which is inserted into the temporal artery located on the side of the baby's wrist, is used instead. Both a UAC and a RAC are used to give infusions and medications or to take blood for blood-gas tests. Such tests are made to analyze the level of oxygen in the blood. Test results help doctors determine the correct level of oxygen the baby needs. The reason that the oxygen level is monitored so carefully is that the baby's eyes, like other parts of the body, are still growing and can be damaged by oxygen. In earlier times, doctors were unaware of the damaging effect of too much oxygen, and many babies were blinded in the process of being saved.

While new medical procedures and equipment are developed almost constantly, it usually takes some time before use of such procedures and equipment is common practice. At this time, three interesting new pieces of equipment are being used in a few neonatal nurseries:

- A nasal cannula, which is a two-pronged, snap-on addition to an oxygen tube, fits into the nose and allows an infant to be taken out of an oxygen hood to be held or breast-fed while still receiving oxygen.
- A tc-pO$_2$ (transcutaneous oxygen) sensor is a nickel-size device that can be taped to an infant's chest to provide a safe, continuous monitoring of the oxygen level of the infant's blood. When used, this sensor replaces the need for repeated blood-gas tests.
- Specially designed waterbeds have been found helpful for premies who have frequent apnea spells. The gentle movements of the waterbed have been shown to decrease the number of apnea episodes.

STAFF

It is also important for parents to know about the nursery staff:

- A neonatologist is a doctor with special training to care for newborns.
- A neonatology fellow is a doctor who works in the NICU and other special care nurseries to gain on-the-job training in neonatology. A fellow's work is supervised by the neonatologist in charge of the unit.
- A resident, who is a hospital employee, has received an M.D. degree, completed an internship and is continuing with specialized training in a particular medical field. An intern has completed four years of medical school and has received an M.D. degree. Employed by the hospital, the intern works in various hospital units to gain practical experience in the practice of medicine. Residents and interns are known collectively as house officers; they form the house staff.
- The senior staff consists of all the other medical doctors, including private pediatricians and academic teachers affiliated with the hospital.
- An R.N. is a registered nurse, and an L.V.N. is a licensed vocational nurse (in some areas called an L.P.N. or licensed practical nurse). Both have completed nurses' training and have met prescribed standards for licensing in the state in which they practice.
- A neonatal nurse has added experience in the neonatal area.
- A nurse clinician is employed by doctors rather than a hospital and is primarily involved with patient education rather than nursing care.
- A perinatal social worker refers patients to sources of information and counseling services. The designation M.S.W. indicates that the person has a master's degree in social work; A.C.S.W. indicates the person is a member of the Academy of Certified Social Workers.
- Therapists give treatment for different medical problems. In an NICU, parents are most likely to encounter respiratory therapists. Some hospitals assign physical therapists to premie units to stimulate and exercise the

undeveloped muscles of some babies.
- Technicians specialize in the technical details of X rays, laboratory work, maintenance of the equipment used in the nurseries and other hospital services.

HOSPITAL POLICIES

Although the equipment and staff of two hospitals may be similar, the policies of the hospitals, or even of two units within the same hospital, may differ. One mother recalled how she and her husband felt when they encountered conflicting hospital policies:

> On the day I was released from the hospital, [the doctors at the children's hospital] felt that Camille was stable enough to go back to [the hospital of birth], which was closer to our home . . . . They allowed us to transport her ourselves . . . to save ambulance costs (provided we didn't stop for pizza on the way!). When we arrived at [the closer hospital], it was the beginning of a very frustrating experience.
>
> After they got her situated, we were able to go in and see her. We asked if we could hold her and the nurse said no; until they received orders from the doctor, we would not be able to. This seemed strange to me since [we] had just [been] allowed . . . to transfer her in our own car. I tried to understand . . . though it bothered me.
>
> Before we left that night, we were given a list of instructions (including that we would be required to call ahead before we came in). I asked why and the nurse said, "Sometimes it's really hectic back here, and we're too busy for parents."
>
> On about the third day, I was holding her [when a] nurse came in and told me it was time to put her back in the Isolette. I questioned this; I felt she had not been out that long. The nurse persisted . . . so I asked her what it said in the doctor's orders. She shrugged her shoulders and walked out of the room, mumbling that she would allow me five more minutes. She came back in fifteen.

This mother added that the nurses at this hospital seemed to have little understanding of the frustration that many parents of hospitalized babies feel. At the time her baby was born, she began corresponding with a mother in Houston whose own son had been premature:

> About that time, we were receiving letters from [a mother whose premie was born and cared for in Houston]. I had written to her of my frustrations, and I cannot express in words adequately my gratitude for her . . . support. I brought one of her letters to the nursery one day for the nurses to read, hoping that they could see what was going on in the world around them, but I just heard excuses such as "Well, we're just not set up for that here."
>
> Also, one time I brought in a very small wind-up lamb to put in the Isolette. They wouldn't let me and couldn't come up with any explanation of why except that "we just don't do that sort of thing here."
>
> Finally, when Camille was twenty-three days old, she was allowed to come home. A long-awaited day had arrived . . . . I brought in the darling premie outfit my friend had sent me. I explained to the head nurse . . . what [my friend] had written me about the many hospitals that encourage [parents] to dress [their] baby [while] in the hospital . . . . She turned to me and said, "You mean you would really bother with that? Think of all the laundry you'd have to keep up with!" Obviously, she missed the entire point.

OTHER SERVICES

Parents of babies in special care nurseries often need to deal with other hospital departments and services, including the admissions office, the labor and delivery unit, the business office and, occasionally, the social services department and the hospital clergy.

Admissions Office

With any impending delivery, the mother must first be admitted to the hospital. Forms requiring information about the patient, insurance companies and policy numbers must be filled out. Since the bill for an infant's intensive care can be several thousand dollars a week, it is important that complete insurance information be provided as quickly as possible to avoid confusion in billing and any unnecessary worry about finances.

Upon admission, a choice must be made between a private and a semiprivate room for the mother after the delivery. If possible, it is wise for the mother who delivers early to be in a private room, or at least in a room with another mother who has had her baby prematurely. The emotional trauma of having a newborn in an NICU is often heightened by being in a room with another mother whose healthy, term baby is brought to her for feedings.

Privacy is important at this time, too. In a private room, parents can deal with this crisis alone and make telephone calls to relatives and friends. Mothers learning to use a breast pump find that pumping is generally easier if done in private. In addition, a husband may wish to stay with his wife; in some hospitals this is permitted only if a patient has a private room.

Some mothers, however, feel that the presence and support of another person in a semiprivate room is comforting.

Occasionally, a doctor may feel that a baby should be transferred to another hospital. This may be due to the severity or unusual nature of the infant's illness or complications or to other factors. Parents of a transfer baby have to deal with more than one admissions office. The mother of one premie and the father of another commented:

> To parents with the heartache and subdued comfort of having to admit their premature infant to the massive buildings and complexity of a giant medical center, this necessary priority—the admissions office—seems unnecessary and somewhat cold and uninviting. Your anxieties for your infant, your loved one, being so sick as to require the help that a medical center can provide, are distant from the business of the situation.

Charlie was transferred . . . . [and when I arrived at the other hospital], I had no idea where to go or what to do. Finally after being sent from [one place to another], I found the emergency admitting room. They told me he was being cared for and to please fill out some forms. I could have cared less about their damn forms. After completing them, I was sent to the NICU [to see my son].

Labor and Delivery Unit

"We intended to go Lamaze and never got a chance to attend a class." This is a common statement of first-time parents whose baby is born too early. Parents of premature babies are faced with the fact that quick decisions must be made about the delivery, and they consequently may have little choice in the way the delivery is handled.

Often, a baby is monitored while the mother is in labor to watch for any sudden changes in the heart rate that may indicate fetal distress. The external fetal monitor, similar to a belt, is placed across the mother's abdomen. In cases where closer monitoring is needed, an internal monitor may be used. A small electrode attached by a wire to the monitor is inserted inside the mother's vagina and attached to the infant's scalp. When a mother is not prepared for use of the monitor, the situation can be distressing.

The presence of a number of unfamiliar doctors and nurses may also be distressing. Although an obstetrician is generally in charge of the delivery, a neonatologist or a pediatrician may also be in the delivery room to care for the baby from the moment of birth. If a mother is transferred to a hospital with a Level II or III nursery, another obstetrician or a resident may deliver the baby.

Because prematurity is considered a complication of pregnancy, husbands who have attended prepared childbirth classes with their wives are sometimes not allowed in the delivery room. Hospital policy and the doctor's assessment of the situation dictates whether or not the father-to-be is permitted in the delivery room. Even a few moments together can be precious.

I was ten weeks early, I had twins and one was a breech, a total of three complications. I was told that even if my husband had completed the Lamaze classes, he could not have entered the delivery room in our case. The doctor knew what we had intended, however, and allowed him to come into the labor area while I was being prepped.

My husband and I saw our son born. From our vantage point, he looked fine and beautiful. He weighed 4 pounds, ½ ounce. We saw him for a moment before he was placed in an incubator and examined by a neonatologist. We didn't even know what a neonatologist was at the time. The memory of just those few moments together sustained us through the next six weeks.

As they wheeled my wife to her room, they took her bed into the intermediate nursery so she and I could see and touch Charlie together. For a moment, we were a complete family. I knew no one could ever take that moment away from us.

Business Office

The business office of a hospital generally has counselors available to advise parents about their child's hospital bill. It is important to meet and work with a counselor within the first few weeks of a baby's hospitalization since the bill is often large. The average stay for an infant born at thirty-two to thirty-four weeks gestation is eight to twelve weeks, and the resulting hospital bill can easily reach $100,000 or more. Parents with major medical insurance may have to pay only 20 percent of the bill, but in some instances, the parents' portion can reach $20,000 or more. In addition, parents will also receive bills from the obstetrician, the baby's private pediatrician, consulting neonatologists, radiologists, surgeons, anesthesiologists, pediatric ophthalmologists, ambulance services and others who provide care.

The bills associated with a premature birth can seem overwhelming to parents.

With a sick premature infant, the resulting bill seems fictional, beyond reality. The computer printout total seems erroneous and inconceivable . . . . It is only with a reminder of the circumstances that one is able to justify it.

At the $60 a month we could afford, it would take us 12½ years to pay the $9,000 left on our bill after the insurance coverage.

A few days after my baby was discharged, we received a bulky envelope in the mail from the hospital. I thought I must have left some of his clothes in the nursery and they were mailing them to me. Wrong! It was the bill . . . thirty-three pages of it, listing everything from his bed to every thermometer and Pamper he used!

Social Services

If parents have difficulty communicating with the medical staff, handling the burden of the hospital bill, coping with the strains placed on the family by an infant's prolonged hospitalization or dealing with other aspects of this experience, they can request assistance from the social services department of that hospital or from a community social services agency.

Some hospitals charge a fee for consultation with the social worker, while others consider counseling a part of the overall service provided to patients.

Many parents have never before consulted a social worker and do not understand the function of a social services department. One parent writes:

I had never personally dealt with a social worker before and I had a lot of preconceived notions about them. Since I did not know that one was being called in, I was very surprised and confused when she phoned me . . . . I immediately and emphatically told her that her services were not needed or wanted.

She sensed my hostility and asked what I thought social workers did. I answered by saying that social workers deal with people who abuse their children or who are on welfare—and I was neither of these! She laughed and [then] explained that she was called in because we had expressed a desire to take our son home on oxygen.

We met in the nursery and she brought us a lot of useful information, including a complete price list of equipment. We discussed at length the pros and cons of having the oxygen in our home. She gave us such tremendous support. She was extremely easy to talk to and was an excellent listener.

Clergy

The hospital clergy is available to support parents during this trying period. They can provide emotional as well as spiritual support. If parents wish, the hospital clergy can give guidance and support when life or death decisions must be made about their infants. Parents who wish to see a clergyman should request to do so.

Special Services

A hospital may offer other services such as a breast-feeding consultant, a breast-milk bank, special educational series for parents of premature or high-risk infants or a follow-up program for these infants. The hospital may also be affiliated with a parent support group or a developmental center, where a variety of medical and child-development specialists assess the child's physical and emotional development. At such centers, infants and young children are observed for signs of developmental difficulties, so that problems can be identified and corrected as early as possible.

DON'T BE AFRAID TO ASK QUESTIONS

The birth of a premature infant exposes parents to new situations that most have not experienced before. It's a world full of unknown doctors, ominous-looking equipment and strange smells and sounds. In the middle of it

all is a son or daughter who belongs to you. The first
things that parents want to and should know are "What
is being done for my baby?" and "Why?" Do not be afraid
to ask questions at any time!

For parents of newly born premies, the last sentence of this
quotation from the mother of a baby girl who weighed 1 pound
15 ounces at birth is one worth remembering.

Communication between parents and the hospital staff is of the
utmost importance. Parents' understanding of or lack of knowledge about their child's problems and possible consequences can
have long-range effects on how parents relate to, react to and
deal with their child.

"What's Going On?"

Communication is always difficult between a professional and
those unfamiliar with the specialized language of that professional's field. Such communication is even more complicated
when it deals with such an emotional issue as the health of a child.
Confusion can arise when the professionals caring for the child
do not agree.

One mother and father whose son was born in Houston in 1976
were told that he had an intraventricular hemorrhage (IVH) and
that he would probably be brain damaged. A CAT scan was not
available at that time in that hospital, and existing methods of
testing were not totally conclusive. The parents asked what this
meant in terms of their son's future. The private pediatrician felt
that the child could either have severe damage or simply be
affected enough to become a "B" rather than an "A" student in
school. A neonatologist felt that the parents should be prepared
for the worst and in a conference with the parents made it clear
that severe brain damage was highly possible. On the basis of
observing the child, the nurse in charge of the NICU privately
disagreed with the bleak prognosis of the neonatologist and let
the parents know that she had seen no extreme abnormalities in
the child's behavior.

How do parents react to such a conflict of opinions? The debate concerns *their* child, whom they want to live, grow and thrive. In this particular case, the parents' emotions swayed each time they heard a new report: from a hopeful "wait-and-see" attitude, to guilt and sadness at the thought of the things their son may never be able to do, to renewed hope when presented with a brighter outlook.

These parents realized that a matter of judgment was involved and that they should keep asking questions. The doctors who care for premies are faced with life-and-death situations on a daily basis, but the questions that arise change as smaller and smaller babies are helped to survive. A doctor may not know whether a baby can be saved nor the possible long-term effects that may result from that baby's early birth. The doctor can only use past experience to deal with the complications that arise. The doctor has a responsibility to the child to follow the course that seems most logical in the treatment of a particular condition. Parents have the responsibility to continually ask questions about treatment which seems incomplete or inadequate. In some instances, parents may wish to seek second and even third opinions from other medical specialists. As one parent puts it:

> The whole thing boils down to the fact that these doctors bust their butts while having to shoot in the dark. They have to make educated guesses based on a hell of a lot of experience and the available facts. But doctors still are not prophets who predict the absolute future. If your child makes it and how well depends to a great extent on how hard your child is willing to fight to live.

Quite often, no one doctor is completely right and no prognosis is completely wrong. Continual reassessment of the situation is called for.

"But I Don't Know What to Ask!"

This complaint is a common one expressed by parents. Most parents are not medically trained, and many have never had a premature infant. They are totally unaware of the procedures, terminology and equipment involved in the saving of these smallest of human lives. As a result, parents often feel they have no idea of what to ask doctors other than "Will our baby live?" "Will our child be normal?" In order to ask pertinent questions, parents must be over the initial shock that may accompany an early birth, and they must have at least some knowledge and understanding of the situation.

Parents who are hesitant about asking questions should remember:

1. *Doctors, nurses and social workers are available to answer any questions.* In one sense, answering questions is part of the job for which they are paid.
2. *No question is unimportant.* Anything that hinders a parent's understanding of the situation is important. A lack of information may be frustrating. Being given too much information all at once can lead to confusion and increased anxiety. At times, words may not be enough. If necessary, parents should ask doctors to draw them simple diagrams to explain a particular medical problem or treatment.
3. *Parents should ask questions for the good of their child.* It is of the utmost importance that parents know about possible complications of their child's prematurity, the probability of a particular problem recurring and any possible long-lasting effects from the medical problems and treatments that their child has had.

One mother recalled how little she knew about prematurity when her baby was born eight weeks early:

I never really concerned myself with prematurity, its causes or its consequences. Even as I sat in my OB's office while I was in premature labor and he expressed concern about the baby's potential problems due to early arrival, I didn't really grasp the fact that those could and would be *our* problems. My husband and I felt as though we were suffering from "jet lag" or "future shock." Things were happening so fast and not as we had planned or expected.

HANDLING FINANCIAL MATTERS AND STRESS

A Professional's Viewpoint

The medical bills of a prematurely born infant are often staggering. At present, there is no funding specifically for prematurity. However, funds for a premie with a long-term disability may be available from federal government programs such as Supplemental Security Income (SSI) and the Women-Infant-Children (WIC) program. To learn more about these programs, ask the hospital's social services department about which federal agency to contact.

Parents whose infants have specific birth defects such as heart defects, cleft lip and palate or other physical handicaps (hearing loss, sight impairment, cystic fibrosis, etc.) may receive assistance from SSI, Crippled Children's Services, national birth-defect foundations or other health-related organizations. For more information, contact a social worker, the local March of Dimes chapter or a local children's information and referral agency. Check also with your state health department; some states have insurance assistance programs for which you may be eligible.

The first step in attacking a large hospital bill is to work with the hospital business office. Get to know the business office staff personally; they'll work with you when they know you. You can usually make arrangements to pay the hospital and doctor's bills on a monthly basis.

Other suggestions for finding funds include bank loans, second jobs, even fund-raising projects by local organizations. Remember, too, that you are not alone in your situation. The priority is your baby's health; the bills will eventually be taken care of.

A Parent's Viewpoint

In attacking your bills, take several initial steps:

1. First, make sure each billing department has complete insurance information: the insurance company's name, policyholder's name, policy number,

special insurance forms if required, mailing address of your insurance company's claims department, names of insurance personnel handling your file if known, etc.

2. Contact your insurance company's claims department to introduce yourself and explain the situation to the person handling your files and/or claims: Give names of hospitals and doctors involved. Keep records of what you discussed, including the names of the insurance personnel you talked with. Occasional calls to persons processing your paperwork can sometimes eliminate delays caused by details such as missing signatures or social security numbers. In contacting any business office, keep in mind that you are not the only person needing their services. Organize your thoughts and questions before calling.

3. Organize bills! You can separate and group them according to hospitals, doctors or services. Keep continuous records on bills and payments posted in a spiral notebook, on the outside of a large envelope containing groups of bills or in some other manner.

4. Contact the billing department of each creditor to whom you owe money. Make them aware of your circumstances and the manner in which you intend to pay. They can note this on your file. Make no promises you cannot keep. Contact them about overdue payments before they contact you. Keep in mind, however, that some creditors will not accept partial payments.

5. Pay off small bills first, while making payments on large, long-term bills. This eliminates the large number of bills received each month and gives the sense of accomplishment that something "has been paid off." As small bills are eliminated, increase payments on larger bills accordingly.

6. For ease in completing income tax forms, keep a separate list of payments on medical bills; include date, check number, recipient, and amount paid.

7. If for any reason your account is turned over to a collection agency, contact the agency as soon as possible and try politely to straighten out any misunder-

standing. Should the discussion become harassing or threatening, remind the agency you have legal protection as a consumer from such threats. If harassment continues, consult a lawyer.

Chapter 3

SHARING COMMON FEELINGS

Few parents initially realize the potentially serious consequences of a premature delivery. But for all, the early birth and prolonged hospitalization bring forth a flood of feelings—some positive, many negative.

> Although my cramping continued, I was too groggy from the Demerol to think right . . . . At 5:30 a.m., a nurse . . . came to check on me. When I sat up to tell her I was still cramping . . . my water broke. She and I were both shocked . . . . I was particularly horrified to observe what I . . . heard labeled "meconium stain." [But] I never considered what might happen to a baby born 2½ months early. Instead, all I could think of was how I wasn't ready to be a mother. We hadn't begun working on the nursery. I had only worn my new maternity outfits once or twice. My students at school wouldn't understand. It was our weekend to shop for the vegetable co-op. We hadn't completed our Lamaze course and we didn't have a pediatrician! Never once did I consider that our baby might not make it.

There he lies, my baby, my little boy. The baby I have hoped for since the . . . days I played mommy with my dolls. Each breath he takes is an effort.

Why has this happened to me? This is an insulting way for my child to begin his life, for me to begin . . . motherhood.

I was the perfect pregnant woman . . . everything in my favor until this nightmare of unexpected labor and delivery at 5½ months.

Will he live? I have never even heard of a baby being born alive at 1½ pounds, let alone living a normal life. There he lies, an IV in his shaved head . . . UAC in his stomach; his legs so severely bruised from birth that they are purple; his legs and arms tied with gauze to the table; 1½ pounds and only 12 inches long.

Will God give us the gift of parenthood? It is as if He has not made up His mind. One day [our son] is fine, the next day he is not; two steps forward, one step back. I'm desperate to be a mother to my own child.

To say precisely how anyone will react to a premature birth is impossible. Each pregnancy and birth is different; each person is unique. An individual's personality, past experiences in life and relationships with others will affect the person's emotional response to a premature birth. How ill the baby actually is and how ill the parents *think* the baby is will likewise influence reactions to the situation.

In general, however, an early birth does create a situation in which hope constantly competes with fear, and altered expectations interfere with the joy of childbirth.

JOY, THEN . . . FEAR

For couples who have suffered through troubled pregnancies, the first feelings after a live birth are often ones of relief or thankfulness.

"I'm not pregnant any more!" That was the first positive feeling I had after Bonni was born thirteen weeks prematurely. It had been a very long pregnancy, topped off by my being confined to bed. I felt now that my own physical problems were over. It was time . . . to get my life back to normal.

The first thing I remember was waking and seeing a clock. I knew I had delivered my baby. Why did I still feel so bad? Why were doctors and nurses everywhere? I was supposed to be fine.

I later found out that I had been unconscious through two critical days, which sometimes happens following a toxemic delivery. . . . I remember asking about my baby. I thought she weighed 4 pounds. Later, I learned she weighed only 2 pounds. My only thought at the time was "Thank God, she's alive."

Even when parents are elated that the child has survived the rigors of birth, many subsequently find themselves torn by emotions. While they may be hopeful that the baby will survive and do well, they may also feel anxious and guilty. Feelings of helplessness and insecurity may develop. Parents may also be resentful, angry or jealous of others. They often believe that they have been rejected by society or that they are somehow failures. Some come to deny or ignore the facts. At one point or another, most feel frustrated, depressed and sad as a result of the fear that accompanies the hope in this crisis.

ANXIETY

Parents unfamiliar with the type of care premies receive or the outcomes of prematurity can become anxious about aspects of hospitalization that are, in fact, not alarming:

Pauline's entire hospital stay was a continual series of ups and downs for us. Some feelings were well-founded, while others were over minor things.

We worried about the oxygen level being lowered and then raised again . . . the IVs in her head . . . the wheezing we felt when holding her . . . her transfer from [one hospital] back to the hospital [where] she was born . . . her inching down out of the oxygen hood . . . not being told everything . . . her pulling at her gavage tube and heart-monitor clips . . . her [N/G] tube . . . becoming dislodged . . . the raising and lowering of cc's of milk given her . . . her activity making it difficult to keep IVs in . . . the return to an IV after being off it . . . her pulling at the bandage over an abscess . . . [the possibility of] the abscess causing brain damage and many other things.

A high level of anxiety makes it difficult for parents to see their baby as a unique person. I saw all the machinery that he was hooked up to, the heaving of his chest as he struggled to breathe and how very skinny he was—but I didn't really see *him.*

Anxiety often results from a lack of information. If parents are concerned or confused, they should question the doctors and nurses caring for their child or seek assistance from the perinatal social worker. In some intances, though, the only honest answer to a question maybe "we just do not know."

GUILT

It is completely logical that an unpredictable, high-risk situation causes extreme anxiety. With a premature delivery, an emotion that is surprisingly often connected with that anxiety is guilt.

"Why is the baby early?" "What will happen to my baby?" When parents ask these questions in their endless variations and the medical professionals whom they ask cannot give definite answers, anxiety builds. In an attempt to find answers where there may not be any, parents frequently direct questions at themselves: "What did I do wrong to cause my baby to come early?" "What problems will my child have as a result of what I did?"

Parents, and mothers in particular, may feel only a momentary sense of guilt or be so overwhelmed by it that they are temporarily incapable of relating to their infants. Here are some common reactions:

An hour later, . . . the reality of our son's serious condition crashed around me . . . . Our private pediatrician, and a neonatologist neither of whom I'd never met before, came to my room. So began the endless words and phrases, the explanations, the noncommitted answers, the negative percentages and the names of the monsters that threatened my baby's lungs, heart, brain and life.

Why hadn't I gone to the hospital immediately? Why did I wait? How could I be so stupid and irresponsible?

I threw stones of guilt at myself. I was the guilty one. I didn't deserve a baby. My baby. I longed to have him back inside of me.

I tried desperately to be brave. I caressed Ryan's little fingers, stroked his little head. Then I was left alone with him for a couple of minutes. I could be brave no more. I looked at him and sobbed, "Oh, baby, what have I done to you? What in God's name did I do wrong?"

I started dreading going to . . . see Bobby; it hurt so much to leave him. . . . Yet I had guilt feelings because I felt I was pushing my baby away by feeling that way. . . . I would be up one minute and down the next . . . . I felt guilty since God has blessed us. Bobby was fine, but I felt cheated. Everyone else had their babies . . . . Why couldn't I be normal? Then the guilt would set in . . . again and I would realize I had a blessing all the money on earth couldn't touch . . . . I was like a seesaw. You become weak from so much emotion, then wake up and start it all over the next day.

Because guilt is one emotion to which parents do not readily admit, many are surprised and comforted to learn how common it is. Most mothers come to feel as one who reflected, "Guilt mellows out when you realize you did all you could while you were pregnant."

At some point, parents are faced with the realization that the "picture-perfect" world they once envisioned during the pregnancy is no longer within their grasp. The feeling that the situation is "less than perfect" or out of their control can cause continued anxiety and guilt about the child's future. But clinging to guilty feelings is not helpful or wise. Infants born at term can also have medical or developmental problems, both at birth and later in life. At any rate, what has been done in the past cannot be changed. Families must look to the future. Says one parent:

> The best advice I could give parents who feel guilty is this: Give up your feelings as soon as possible. Feeling guilty will not help your child; being a concerned, loving parent will.

HELPLESSNESS

Faced with a tiny infant in an incubator, a parent may feel deprived of the responsibilities of parenthood. A feeling of helplessness results as parents realize they cannot care for their own child as well as the hospital staff can. Mothers who feel a strong maternal instinct may be particularly upset.

> I had a very sick premie and what could I do about it? It was obvious that I had no magic spell or new miracle cure, so just what could I contribute to his recovery? I felt like I was in the way at times . . . . I felt so useless and inadequate.

A strong maternal instinct does not always develop immediately. One mother who did not want to see or name her baby after birth said:

> I guess I thought if I had no contact, it wouldn't matter if she died. The [doctors] finally convinced me [to see her], but I felt nothing when I looked at her.
>
> When I was released from the hospital, I went to [the transfer hospital], took one look and threw up. She was so ugly—she looked like a freak (which was something I couldn't, and didn't, admit to myself until a couple of years after her birth). I felt desperation, fear, panic—and a feeling of helplessness.

Mothers are not the only ones who feel helpless. One father who accompanied one of his twin sons to another hospital in an ambulance was caught in traffic at a critical time. His wife related the story:

> Steve had worked in an ambulance when he was younger, but he said this was the worst ride of his life. They were in five o'clock traffic . . . only going seven miles, yet cars wouldn't get out of the way.
>
> Two ladies blocking the lane ahead sat in their car talking, ignoring the siren. Steve said he wanted to kill them. The ambulance driver finally bumped the car to get their attention and they moved. By the time the ambulance pulled into . . . emergency, Steve glanced at Dunc and saw he was blue.
>
> The baby was whisked upstairs and Steve followed at breakneck speed. An admitting clerk tried to stop him. He told her to go to hell, he'd be back later.
>
> After Dunc was stabilized, the neonatology fellow talked to Steve and answered all the questions that he could. Our biggest question, "Will he live?" was unanswerable.
>
> Steve came back to see me but sat outside the room until he was in control enough to come in. He stayed with me awhile and then home to try to rest.
>
> I think the heaviest burden is . . . on the daddies. They think they have to be brave for our sakes . . . . It's so hard on them when they're afraid, too.

INSECURITY

Even experienced parents often feel insecure about caring for their infant and are intimidated by not being able to talk to or hold their infants without a nurse or doctor hovering nearby. At home their insecurity becomes even worse:

> When your baby comes home, you know it's up to you twenty-four hours a day. I lay awake many nights frequently checking to see if the twins were still breathing.
>
> I wanted the boys home but doubted my ability to care

for them as well as the hospital personnel. Only recently have I gotten over the feeling that medical authorities have the last say over what I can or cannot do with my own children.

Parents whose baby has had many medical problems are particularly vulnerable to feelings of insecurity.

It is with a certain amount of embarrassment that I talk about the heart monitor.

From the day Victor was born . . . he was on a heart monitor. And for nearly four months, his monitor alarm [sounded] constantly. It was only the last two weeks of Victor's hospital stay that we didn't hear or hear *of* numerous alarms. So when we were told that Victor could go home, I knew we would rent a heart monitor. Facing Victor without one was unthinkable.

It wasn't easy finding one. It wasn't cheap, either . . . . We located one . . . the morning of the day that Victor was discharged. The hospital doctors refused to sign the order . . . that was necessary to obtain a monitor. They deemed it "medically unnecessary."

Thrilled as we were over Victor's recovery, I guess I just couldn't immediately erase the awful picture burned into my mind of Victor during one of his spells.

We contacted Victor's neurologist and explained our predicament to him. He willingly signed the prescription. I don't mean to imply he thought *Victor* needed a monitor. But I'm sure he understood how much *we* needed it.

A certain amount of insecurity is a normal by-product of anxiety and other stresses. It is not uncommon for parents to think that their child "must be pretty sick if he's on a heart monitor" and then be concerned when the monitor is removed. Although the removal of the monitor is an indication that the child's health has improved, the parent misses the security of the machine's constant guardianship.

Caring for the baby in whatever ways permitted during the child's hospitalization can be helpful in reducing later insecurity. With practical experience comes self-confidence. One mother admitted that she had never expressed her self-doubts aloud or even to herself, until a perceptive friend remarked, "Don't worry. You can take care of that baby just fine."

RESENTMENT, JEALOUSY AND ANGER

Parents may also feel angry at or jealous of the nurses who give such loving care to their babies. One mother writes:

> One day I was making my afternoon visit when a pregnant nurse told me it was time to leave, then took my baby from my arms and sat down to rock him.
>
> "I could rock him," I thought. "What difference would it make if I stayed and rocked him instead of her? He's my baby. They act like I'm not his mother, that I'm not capable of doing even simple things for him."
>
> I was angry when I left the hospital that afternoon. I resented the nurse who took my baby away from me. But most of all, I was jealous of the time she had to hold and touch him.
>
> Two days later, he was all mine and those feelings slowly melted away into a grateful memory of the wonderful nursing care my son received.

Anger, a result of helplessness, fear and guilt, is not always directed only at the medical staff, but often at oneself as well. Parents may find themselves angry at their child, too, for being the source of such stress.

The inability to change or control specific policies, events or circumstances is frustrating. Many parents, for example, come to resent the lack of privacy in most nurseries.

> Even though the nurses were kind and the nurseries were open to parents, there was a very un-private air in the nursery. One day I sat arm against arm with another mother . . . jabbering sweet nothings to my daughter as the other mother did the same . . . with the nurses leaning over us to add their sweet comments.
>
> I thought, "My God, we're mother apes in cages, and

they are all waiting to spring in case we don't get along with our babies."

CONFUSION

Parents bombarded by medical information can become confused. Sometimes they feel so lost in the maze of terminology that they do not know how to phrase questions or even what to ask. In extreme cases, they may completely stop asking for information about their infant. In some instances, the information given to parents is not as complete as it should be.

> Two days after my daughter's surgery for necrotizing enterocolitis, we were awakened by a call from the hospital asking us to come immediately and give permission for another operation. We had no idea why she needed a second operation and were quite disconcerted until a doctor explained that the placement of the catheter for transparenteral hyperalimentation required a surgical procedure.
>
> We had been informed the day before about the catheter, but it had been explained to us in simplified terms by a nurse—as a tube. Not once had anyone used the words "surgery" or "operation." Not being "medical people," we just didn't realize what putting a catheter in a baby physically entailed.

Confusion caused by incomplete information is best alleviated by answers. Unfortunately, misunderstood answers often lead to more confusion. To understand the situation, parents may wish to make a list of their child's problems, what they mean and what the doctors intend to do about them. Confusion can also be a result of stress. Answers are more easily understood by a parent who is receptive to listening.

There is confusion of another sort, too. Do parents send out birth announcements? If so, when? Does the father pass out cigars? Should baby showers that had been planned be canceled?

Ryan's parents decided to send out birth announcements soon after his birth, but not without some moments of indecision:

At four days of age, Ryan was in grave condition. We really didn't know if he would survive. Yet I desperately longed to let the whole world know that he had arrived.

Should we send out birth announcements or not? My husband and I went back and forth, back and forth.

Finally he said, "Let's send them. After all, you did give birth to him and that's what we are announcing."

REJECTION AND FAILURE

Parents of a premature infant may feel rejected by society. Their babies are objects of curiosity to hospital nursery visitors. Even relatives and friends often do not know what to say or do. These parents have "failed" to produce a baby that carries society's stamp of approval.

During our baby's fourth week in the hospital, my husband and I became more confident that he would survive. This new self-assurance and hope sparked a sense of pride and a great parental desire to show off our first child, so we asked friends to come to the hospital to see our son.

We had adjusted to our baby's small size and the sights and sounds of a premature nursery, but many of our friends were shocked or overwhelmed. We were disappointed, angered and sometimes hurt by their response or lack of response.

It's easy now to look back and try to understand and forgive them for their fears. If you've not been in the same situation yourself, it must seem peculiar to watch two smiling parents holding their "abnormal-looking" baby up to the window for your admiration. After all, what do you say to them? The usual new baby comments are out of place. You certainly can't say how big, fat and healthy the baby is. There are no pretty praises for the baby hair that has been shaved off in patches and strips for IVs. How can you say he looks just like either parent?

I sent out birth announcements [while] I was still in the hospital. No one wrote back—no cards—no gifts—just some flowers from close, local friends. I was crushed. No one acknowledged [her birth].

Mothers may feel special disappointment that the pregnancy has ended. Often, they feel cheated of the total experience of carrying and bearing a child; they may consider themselves to be failures at being pregnant.

> At first, I felt that if Charlie had been born to a "normal" woman she could have carried him to term. I had a mixed-up notion that carrying a baby to term made a good mother . . . . I felt like such a failure as a person and as a mother. Millions of women have perfectly normal pregnancies and very routine deliveries. I had neither of these.

Most parents appreciate relatives and friends who celebrate the baby's birth in some tangible way—a telephone call, card, gift —and offer realistic words of hope and encouragement. Valued most of all are those who are available to listen when parents need to talk.

Strangers, who in a sense represent society as a whole, can also give comfort and hope to parents. One Houston paramedic will never be forgotten by Trey's parents. As their son was being transferred and as his parents stood by anxiously, this stranger said to them, "That's a fine son you have there." These simple words gave that couple renewed hope and strength to face the days ahead.

Contact with local support groups specifically for parents of premature infants can also assist parents in coping with a premature birth. Those who have firsthand knowledge of the experience can give parents more realistic support and encouragement than others may be able to offer.

DENIAL AND DISBELIEF

Some parents ignore statements they do not want to accept or refuse to make logical conclusions based on facts.

When Victor had been in the infant care unit for a week, I met a doctor who held out little, if any, hope for him. The resident pronounced, at our first meeting, that babies with Victor's problem usually never sit up, walk or talk.

"If he manages to live, he'll be a vegetable; he'll have to be institutionalized." He repeated this on more than one occasion.

Each time I heard it, I just got deafer . . . . [Finally], I ceased to hear him.

The first time he said it to me, I fought back tears. I felt like I'd been personally attacked. I'd never heard *anything* so awful. But I made up my mind that these were only words.

[*Editor's note:* At the age of 13½ months, Victor, who was born at twenty-four to twenty-six weeks gestation, functions like a 6½-month-old; but his parents report that he sits and "socializes beautifully" and is making progress.]

One day in the third week, Tommy had a relapse. He was blue almost my entire visit and needed oxygen several times. I couldn't believe it. Everything [had been] going so well. This caught me off guard. I cried for hours uncontrollably. I hadn't realized that he could still die. I was emotionally exhausted and considered seeking professional help. My husband contacted the nurse in charge of the neonatal unit and she spoke with me. Progress began . . . but I never let my guard down again.

When medical complications arise, parents of premies are often stunned. They must confront the feeling that "this couldn't possibly be happening." They also need to analyze any overly optimistic reactions when their child is having serious difficulties. This is not to say that parents should lose hope, only that they should try to approach all facts realistically.

FRUSTRATION AND DEPRESSION

Mothers of premies may feel the "baby blues" more sharply than mothers of term infants due to stress and separation. Fathers may be depressed by the financial obligations that result, frustrated with the realization that the family savings may be wiped out totally or that indebtedness may last for years. Both parents may, at times, feel totally defeated by circumstances. Below are some common reactions:

> I tried to be a little trooper. I thought we wouldn't be treated as well if I acted like a typical, upset mother, so I didn't. One resident told me about Dunc's PDA. I asked if he could die from it (his RDS was finally getting better), and she said yes. I thought I would faint and had to sit down. As soon as she left, the nurse told me his PDA was minor . . . . I felt better but wanted to leave right away so I could cry. That was one of the first of the ups and downs. Every time one thing would improve, something else would get worse.

> I got to touch Aimee as they brought her from the operating room. All I remember seeing is the mass of tubes attached to her and her tiny, tiny arms and legs. I got to see her one more time before the transport team took her to [the children's hospital]. Her fragility, helplessness and smallness left a deep impression and then I realized how much I feared for her.
> I cannot recall much of what else occurred during the next four days . . . . I remember being afraid to call [the children's hospital] for several reasons. One is the obvious one that I was afraid to hear bad news. Secondly, I just couldn't concentrate on what was explained to me . . . . I just couldn't comprehend it. I felt totally overwhelmed by the whole situation.
> If something negative was said, I took it personally and felt responsible for the situation. Several times, I was asked by different nurses when I was going to visit Aimee. I didn't understand why they asked, as I was incapacitated [by my Cesarean section]. Then I conjured

up the idea that the nurses thought I was avoiding them, Aimee and the hospital purposely.

One night we went in for our visit and they had [our daughter's] arms and legs pinned down. She had an IV in her right foot and a transfusion in her left hand. She was twisting and squirming and crying. She cried the whole 1½ hours we were there, and I cried all the way home and after.

I knew she had to have these and would pull them out if not pinned down, but it still hurt me to see her so uncomfortable. I wanted to pick her up and comfort her, but I couldn't. All I could do was sit and watch her struggle to get loose. That was the worst thing I had to see [during her entire hospital stay]!

Frustration and depression, like all the other emotions commonly experienced by parents of premies, can be normal reactions to extreme stress. If a mother's depression is so severe that it becomes postpartum psychosis, she needs medical treatment. If depression is a side effect of the often wildly fluctuating emotions, the parent may need time, emotional support and possibly some professional counseling to weather the crisis.

GRIEF AND SORROW

Currently, approximately 10 percent of the infants born weighing less than 5½ pounds die. Often, those who survive brush close enough to death that their parents must face its reality, sometimes for the first time in their lives.

Many of us in the baby-making stage of our lives have not experienced the death of a loved one so close to us.

The death of a baby seems so unfair. Expectant parents spend months moving everything around in their lives to make room for the new family member. If the baby doesn't arrive as planned, it leaves a big empty hole in your life and your heart.

Every parent whose baby develops one or more of the life-threatening complications of prematurity must at some point acknowledge the possibility of death. Facing the fact that a baby may die is an awesome, awful burden, for babies are not only unique individuals but also, in many ways, extensions of their parents. Some parents avoid confronting the possibility; others find calm after confronting the fear.

> Every time I look at [my son's] face today, I remember how I sometimes avoided it. Not that he had an unattractive face, for he had, and still does have, an angel's face. But often when I looked down at that beautiful little face, I wondered, "Is this the last time?" I just didn't want to be forever haunted by that angelic little face if he had died. Strange how we defend our weaknesses.

> As I waited for my husband [to return from the transfer hospital], my mind filled with thoughts: "What did our minister say that Sunday several months ago about Dr. Elisabeth Kubler-Ross and her research with clinically dead patients who had been revived? . . . They all reported to her that a dead friend or loved one welcomed them into an 'afterlife.'
>
> "If that is true, who will be there for Susan if she dies? . . . Of course! My father—her grandfather, who would have loved her dearly if he were still alive. And Tim's grandfather; he would get to see his first great-grandchild after all . . . . Well, at least she'll be among those who love her as much as I do."
>
> For some reason, a strange calm replaced the great fear I had felt. Just why, I don't know.

There is also extreme disappointment that events have gone awry; hopes and dreams have vanished.

> Cry I did for a while, little Scotty more than holding his own within his pretend placenta. So heartbreaking for me to see medicine's answer for my body . . . . Wishing futilely he was back within me, I already miss his timely kicks . . . . Scotty is handed to me . . . . I feel as though I'm grasping a bundle of air. And again I feel the tears

come. Scotty, I'm so wordlessly sorry, so overwhelmed at
your early arrival.

Some parents "mourn the lost child" of their dreams. The loss
of their "dream" child may have a powerful effect on parents of
premies. A premie is not the full-cheeked "Gerber" baby many
parents expect. The baby's undeveloped features and lean, tiny
body can shatter expectations.

COMMON EXPERIENCES AND FEELINGS

Women, particularly, may feel that the pregnancy is somehow
unfinished when birth occurs too early. They sense that something is missing. They say they feel cheated or that they were not
ready emotionally to give birth.

> I was three months along when I was told I was preg-
> nant, then delivered three months later. I didn't have
> enough time to mentally grasp the idea that I was going
> to have a baby. I feel that I only carried for three
> months.

While some women who give birth prematurely are hospitalized prior to delivery and have an idea of what may happen, most
are surprised when labor begins too early. Some say they cannot
believe it, even as they are on their way to a hospital.

> I was scared, but determined not to fall apart. My due
> date was two months away. I called the doctor, and he
> didn't seem overly concerned. He told me I could go to
> the hospital and be checked by a nurse or I could come
> into the office in the morning. After telling him I'd see
> him at the office, . . . I decided to go to the hospital after
> all.
>
> My husband and I thought we'd go and come right
> back . . . . I read about what water breaking meant in
> some pregnancy books on the way to the hospital. I still
> didn't believe what was happening.

For all parents of hospitalized babies, that first visit to the nursery is etched into their memories.

> I looked in on Matt later that evening and was not really prepared for what I saw. Here was my baby lying on a flat table, surrounded by equipment, attached to tubes. No matter how much the neonatologist tried to prepare me during labor, [I was not] prepared. All I could manage were a lot of tears. I was encouraged to touch him. Where?

Karen's mother was heavily sedated with alcohol during delivery and afterwards could not be awakened to see her daughter before the baby was transferred:

> Strangely enough, it was like not even having a baby at all. Three days after her birth, my husband drove me to the hospital. I had to take a long wheelchair ride from the emergency room to the intensive care nursery. It seemed like an eternity to me.
>
> My first impression of the baby was that she was smaller than the pictures really showed and that she was beautiful. After a moment's observation, we came to the conclusion that she looked like my father—no, she looked like a little old man!
>
> I was afraid to touch her and talk to her through the holes in the Isolette as I didn't want to expose her to my germs.

The sense of failure many women feel is often heightened upon the new mother's discharge from the hospital and her arrival home—alone. Said one mother, "Other mothers carried their babies to their cars .... I carried flowers." Another said:

> I had stayed in the hospital an extra day; then, it was time to go. Unceremoniously, I was wheeled to the car. I felt like a failure.
>
> I entered our home sadly. Only the flowers reminded me that this should have been a happy occasion. The

nursery had been readied months before. I was afraid to peer into its emptiness. I was afraid not to. Picking up an oversized teddy bear, my surrogate baby during my pregnancy, I tried to compare it to Zachary's size. He could have lain upon its lap like a baby doll.

Most parents find the hospitalization of their infant a trying period. When babies stay in the nursery for a long time, parents feel growing frustration.

We never thought it would take so long before our baby would be home with us. Matt had many complications . . . . Needless to say, [his] problems were frustrating, not only to us but also to the medical staff . . . . After a while, Matt was the oldest baby in the nursery. Other babies came and went but Matt stayed.

Having a baby in the hospital nursery can be as much work as caring for the baby at home.

Some people think that you have a vacation while your child is in the hospital. I was told how fortunate I was that I didn't have to get up at 2 a.m. for feedings and that I would be so rested by the time the baby got home.

No one thought about the fact that I was pumping my milk with a machine every three or four hours and making two round trips to the hospital a day and still trying to keep up with a two-year-old.

Other children, relatives, friends and strangers can put real strains on parents and their families by criticizing and making unthinking comments.

The birth of a premature child is like a broken promise for the brother or sister who has been waiting for months for the new playmate to arrive.

Sheri went to preschool the day after Bonni was born and told all of her friends about her new tiny baby sister. But the other kids laughed and said no baby could be that small. The next school day Sheri had a phantom stomach-ache . . . . We talked to her and discovered the real reason behind her tummy troubles.

We made arrangements with the hospital for Sheri to see Bonni and then she was sure that her sister was that small. Sheri took pictures of her sister to school and very proudly showed them to her classmates. No one teased her again.

The phone calls came daily, and daily I would feel like screaming, "I don't know! I don't know if being on oxygen will blind him! I don't know how much longer he'll have to be on a respirator! I don't know when I'll be able to hold him, but God, how I long to! I don't know how I can stand it! I don't know how I'm being so strong!" (Am I being so strong?)

These same questions were going through my mind all day and all night but when I had to talk about them with others it was even harder. Aren't mothers *the most knowledgeable ones* about their own infants? Well, no. Not in the case of a sick one. You wish you did have some secret inside information, some maternal ESP.

Like most parents, friends and relatives usually do not know how to deal with the crisis of a premature birth. Often, an unintentional inappropriate remark, action or demeanor is actually a reflection of true concern and caring. Grandparents have been known to tell relatives not to send gifts until the infant is stable or to suggest canceling showers, in an attempt to spare parents more suffering.

THE PARADOX

While primary attention is focused on the baby, parents may feel their babies do not need them or that they are in the way of the doctors and nurses. On a personal level, they feel they have been denied—at least, temporarily—all the joys of parenthood. These parents, who in the happier days of pregnancy may have anticipated the delight of having a new child to love, have no baby to care for, no son or daughter to play with, sing to or show off proudly to visitors. They feel alone.

> We were allowed to bring toys to put in the Isolettes, so we went on a shopping trip and found two identical yellow lions. At home, we wound them up and put them on our coffee table, along with a musical mobile. We both choked up listening to Brahms' Lullaby alone in our living room.
>
> We tried to do for our babies everything that was suggested. We brought booties and pictures and talked to them and stroked them. I wish someone had stroked us. I felt so incompetent and so impotent.

Chapter 4

THE POSITIVE SIDE

Wait a minute! There's more to it than that! All of you are emphasizing the negative things. For us, it was a good experience because our baby lived and I lived. I almost died, and people were so kind and caring for us. It brought out the best in everyone we knew.

It is easy to emphasize the negative aspects of having an infant prematurely. Yet most parents eventually realize that there are positive aspects as well. Parents often are overwhelmed by the support they receive from relatives, friends, the medical staff and even strangers. They also can find true delight in their child. Many discover an inner strength, faith or insight into life that can help them through future everyday crises.

THE GIFT OF KIND HEARTS

For parents, one of the most positive aspects of dealing with the birth of a premature infant, other than the survival of the child, is the aid and support of others.

Medical Staff

The hospital temporarily becomes a second home for some parents. As a result, the actions, reactions, opinions and observations of the medical staff can greatly influence parents' emotions. Many doctors and nurses are exceptionally sensitive and caring. Some parents feel a special attachment to the nurses.

> Anne and Linda, two of the nurses, became our closest contacts in the premature nursery. They talked to us on a personal level and were sensitive to our concerns. They remembered details of our baby's day. One day our son held up a team of cardiologists and a very expensive piece of equipment for twenty minutes until his hiccups subsided. That story made us feel close to the nurses for relating it and made our son seem more like a small person with a personality of his own.

> I wonder if the nurses realize the powerful effect they have. They always seemed so competent and caring. They would . . . [rock] the babies when they had spare time. They were wonderful on the phone . . . and never made me feel like I was in the way.

> As we left, I felt so thankful to . . . all the wonderful, compassionate doctors and nurses who had cared for me and my son . . . . I wanted to hug and thank each one of them. Yet thanks just doesn't seem enough for all they did.

To thank the staff for the work they have done, some parents buy candy, some bring cakes or other baked goods to the nursery, some give small gifts. All know that such tokens and kind thoughts can in no way compensate for the time and skill doctors and nurses have invested in their children.

Family

Families often give parents help by caring for other children, lending money, offering a hand between travels to the hospital, as well as giving emotional support.

My mother stayed at our house taking care of our two-year-old, Lisa. She would stay up at night and crochet hats and booties for the baby. The nurses would let her go in and visit, but she was afraid to hold Sara. The nurses teased her and said, "Oh, no, Granny, you're not getting out of it," and they would wrap Sara up and have her hold her . . . . It was a positive thing for me to have her there.

Susan's [paternal] grandfather surprised me. The day that she was born, he went home from his office, cut one of the prettiest hyacinths in his garden and brought it to me—the woman who had just given birth to his first grandchild much too early.

A little later, after he learned that she could wear clothes in the nursery, he kept insisting that I take measurements; he had already asked a seamstress to make Susan some gowns. A few days after I got all the information together on size, fabrics to use, etc., he brought me six pink gowns, in different sizes, for his granddaughter.

Susan's grandmothers helped, too. My mother-in-law, who is a practical woman, used her position as a hospital volunteer to order, at a discount, from the hospital pharmacy a whole case of Premie Pampers! My mother cooked for us, helped clean our house and gave support for my efforts at breast pumping. Later, when Susan was home, she stopped by every afternoon after work to play with her granddaughter, which gave me time to relax for a few minutes or to get dinner started.

Friends and Strangers

Friends also provide both physical and emotional help. In addition to being ready listeners, friends may care for other children, raise money, provide parents with opportunities for rest and relaxation, offer transportation to the hospital and make premie-size baby clothes. Parents should tell friends exactly what they need and let them know how much their help is appreciated.

Margaret was always there. I could only visit at set fifteen- or thirty-minute visiting periods twice a day, and

I didn't know how to drive. Margaret—or someone—was always there.

Linda and Joe came to the hospital the day Susan was born. They were a source of great comfort to both Tim and me, as we faced our daughter's transfer to another hospital because of breathing difficulties.

Later, our friends took their four children—all of them our godchildren—to the hospital to see our new, tiny daughter from the other side of the nursery window.

On Easter Sunday, we discovered a small basket on top of Susan's Isolette. Included in the basket, left by the "Easter Bunny and friends," was the smallest Holly Hobbie doll I'd ever seen—just the right size for our daughter!

On the day Susan came home, Linda arranged for child care for all her kids and came over to help me in any way I needed. In the months that followed, I called her for advice (nonmedical!) almost as much as I called the pediatrician!

Acquaintances or coworkers may make a special effort to offer encouragement or help in a tangible way.

One of the most uplifting memories of Trey's early days of struggle for life was the unexpected and most generous gift from my husband's coworkers. We received an envelope full of dollar bills—ones, tens and twenties—I do not remember now the total . . . but I do remember it being well over a hundred dollars.

With Trey and me both in the hospital, George had been able to work only a little over half a day for at least two weeks . . . so his checks had become rather small. This envelope filled with greenbacks looked like the pot of gold at the end of the rainbow to us.

We received that envelope a second time . . . . How can you thank such people who reach out with open hearts and kindness, especially when none of those bills had the previous owner's ID stamped on it? I do know we felt their sympathy and treasured their kindness.

Diary entry: August 4—So many people have taken an interest in you. Pam . . . called me tonight to find out how you are doing and to tell me she got two more people to go and donate blood for you. Craig, her husband, has already given . . . . She has also lined up the . . . Fire Department to go and give blood in your name . . . . I've never even met her . . . . It's just amazing.

[*Editor's note:* This mother noted in an earlier diary entry that a group she and her husband belonged to gave a dance and donated the $81 the group collected to the parents.]

Strangers, too, often give unique support. The common bond formed among parents visiting the nurseries often leads to friendships and new perspectives.

While we were a part of the waiting room "neighborhood," we heard the stories of distraught parents: a boy trapped in a refrigerator and still unconscious, a baby girl born without an abdominal wall, a baby with meningitis, a toddler accidentally given too much medication . . . . Listening to the other stories was like therapy. It was the first step toward a perspective of our personal tragedy.

Other Support

Medical, religious, community and other resources play a large part in parents' emotional survival.

I have received support from many different sources within the community, including the parent support group, county public health nurses, doctors, all with the infant stimulation program. All helped to keep our family together and [helped me keep] my sanity. I am very grateful for them and their obviously caring concern.

Other parents describe as invaluable willing listeners or those who go out of their way to say a kind word:

Friday, our senior minister came to see us just as we were leaving to see Will. He told us that [our] little boy had a direct line to God, and he would pull through. How we wanted this!

I developed a very good rapport with one of the nursery social workers. It was so nice to have someone to talk to. I am the type who needs to talk out her feelings and thoughts. The social worker certainly did a lot of listening. I think this was the only way I was able to cope with the situation.

THE GIFT OF NEW LIFE

The delight parents find in their new infants and the intense love felt when parents and child are together produce positive feelings.

Immediately after my release, we went to the intensive care unit at the other hospital to see Twin A. It was as I thought it would be. The nurse put her in my arms—she was so tiny and so helpless. I was a little afraid of pulling the wires loose. As I held her, I told her how much I loved her and said, "Keep fighting; you're going to make it." I sang to her and prayed for her and then I kissed her and went to see her sister. I repeated all of this with her. I hated to leave but was comforted in knowing they were getting the best of care.

Before she was transferred to the [other] hospital, the transport team brought her to me in the recovery room. She was in an Isolette, and even though I didn't get to hold her, those were a few of the most precious moments of my life.

Each improvement in the child's condition becomes a milestone to be celebrated.

Lisha was on oxygen and a respirator for a long, long time
. . . . One of her nurses, and a gal who has become a

wonderful friend as well, called one evening about 10 p.m., and said, "Elisha's been extubated. Come up and see her. She's beautiful." I threw on my coat and ran. The experience of seeing her face, completely, for the first time was one that can't be described.

We called in a neurologist of our own. His were the first positive words we had heard about our baby. He suggested that Victor would "outgrow" his a. and b. [apnea and bradycardia] spells. He couldn't find anything alarmingly wrong with the baby.

On Friday the 13th, Victor had one a. and b. Then— no more. It was too much to hope for. Twenty-four hours with no spells . . . . I can just imagine God saying, "All right, Victor Veillon Hill, you've been here long enough. It's time for you to go home."

Each affirmation of the child's beauty, normalcy or will to live reassures the parents. Responses from the child, opening the eyes or the semblance of a smile, produce emotional peaks that compensate for many of the valleys.

Diary entry: Your dad and I got to hold you for the first time! Once in the afternoon and once at night. You really seemed to like it. They turned the overhead lights out and you really were looking around. Big eyes! I got to kiss you for the first time, too.

THE GIFT OF SELF-GROWTH

A positive outcome of a premature birth is the personal growth parents may achieve. This growth may be felt as increased faith or trust in God, renewed self-confidence or an insight into the needs of others living through a similar crisis.

Having been agnostic, if not atheistic, throughout college, my newfound faith was on shaky ground . . . . But the most important thing I feel I learned from the crisis dealt with the faith that there was someone else in control of the situation. I had always been a very ordered person, for whom control was important.

When you are thrown into a situation where events that occur are so far beyond your control, you are helpless unless you believe that there is a power greater than your own. If you believe that, then you know that all things ultimately happen for a reason. [Then] even death can bring . . . [some] knowledge [or understanding].

Having a premie was the most devastating experience of my life. It affected every aspect of my life and therefore changed me as a person. I believe I have grown in many ways, and as horrid an experience as it seemed at the time, I am able to look back and appreciate the entire episode as a learning process.

I believe very deeply that I love and appreciate my son *more* now because of the supreme effort we both put forth to succeed and emerge from our first few months of trauma than I would have, had he been [born at] term. I credit this experience for my greater appreciation of life.

Self-growth can bring new vision. Parents may begin to see potentially negative aspects of hospitalization in a new way. The technological monsters that at first seemed to intrude are later appreciated as marvels that help keep alive life and hope.

Several parents have found that setbacks can hold surprising advantages.

I just couldn't believe the stroke of bad luck we were having with everything. First having the premature baby and now not being able to visit her, as Alicia [had the chicken pox]. Alicia first became ill . . . after Aimee had . . . been transferred from the Level III ICU nursery at [the children's hospital] to the Level II nursery at the hospital where she was born . . . . So we had something positive on which to fall back.

Even though it was extremely frustrating at the time, it did provide a relief of some sort in that I was forced to slow down a bit and was given the opportunity to "catch my breath" and get a little rest. It also made me realize how much I was neglecting Alicia. We had to reevaluate our priorities and decided that we were being unfair to place Aimee's hospitalization as top priority. Consequently, we tried our hardest to resume [a] family atmosphere once again.

One mother, who had a particularly positive perspective on the experience, offered this advice:

> Try to look positively at everything, even though sometimes the going is rough. I have heard so many mothers lament about how they felt about being dismissed from the hospital [and having] to leave the baby behind. May I share my feelings?
>
> I was thirty-five when my first and only child, a daughter, was born, after I thought I was never going to be able to have a child. Even though I had to leave her . . . at the hospital for six weeks, I rejoiced that she lived, was very healthy . . . . was perfectly formed and was a beautiful child.

RESULTS OF POSITIVE FEELINGS

One of the interesting results of the positive outlook of some parents are the symbolic, late-chosen names of a number of the children. Will was given his name because "he had a will to live." Victor was the only name his mother would consider because "the little baby who faced such insurmountable problems—about whom everyone talked so pessimistically—would be victorious." Matthew means "gift of God." Aimee was "loved."

Perhaps the most apparent result of having a positive attitude is reflected in parents' desire to reach out to other parents. One woman expressed clearly the view held by the parents who contributed to this book:

> It makes me feel . . . good inside to reach out to the women who are in this situation now. If by writing this, it helps one person to feel better, . . . handle the situation better and cope with her own feelings, I have spent my time very beautifully.

Almost all parents of premies are at times filled with great hope. They believe in their baby and the doctors and nurses, in their friends and relatives, in themselves and in the future. That such bright hopes can exist in the midst of a situation where there is such tremendous potential for despair is a tribute to the human spirit. It is evidence of the power of the love that most parents have for their babies.

To Be Happy

Rules for happiness:
Something to do;
Something to love;
Something to hope for.
Immanuel Kant

Chapter 5

THE NEED TO COMMUNICATE

Just a few months before, we were so happy. Everything was going our way. We were expecting our second child, and once he was here, our life would be perfect and complete. Nothing had turned out like we had wanted or expected. We were being pulled from every direction. Charlie had complication after complication. Every time we thought we were over one hurdle, there was another one to take its place.

Like a piece of taffy, a couple going through a crisis feels stretched by a barrage of events and emotions. Forming a relationship with anyone is no easy task; melding a partnership is even more difficult. Deepening the bonds of that partnership while under stress is a challenge of the highest order.

> There is an old saying that you never know what you can handle until you have to. I guess that sums up what Joe and I went through with Joey's premature birth. Our experiences led to a much stronger marriage, and we found a new and deeper meaning to the word "love."

> I heard a beautiful saying during this time: "Patience is love under pressure." Oh, how true!

Together we went through stages of excitement and depression, rejoicing together in our excitement, consoling each other during times of depression. Our lines of communication remained open through the entire ordeal.

The two women whose words are quoted are fortunate. Learning about love and keeping lines of communication open during a crisis are positive goals that a couple can strive for, but in the turmoil of the situation, these goals sometimes seem impossible to achieve.

COMMUNICATION

Emotional and verbal communication between a husband and wife is vital to the survival of a marriage enduring the crisis of premature birth.

To communicate effectively, a couple must not only listen carefully to what is being said aloud but also be observant and attuned to nonverbal language.

Communicating during a crisis requires great effort, patience and understanding at the very time when there may be little patience and understanding to spare.

To relate events, parents must have facts. To share emotions, a husband and wife must be in touch with their own feelings. Most hospital experiences involve a combination of facts and emotions, and the communication concerning both can be clouded by misunderstandings. Moreover, a couple's rapport with each other will be influenced by their rapport with doctors and nurses, family members and friends whose statements can add to emotional strain and complicate communication.

BREAKDOWNS IN COMMUNICATION

Temporary or long-term problems in communication can lead to difficulties in a marriage. The death of a premature infant is an obvious example of a time when channels of communication must remain open or problems can occur.

> After the death of one of our twins, Windy, my husband would only talk about our other twin. He would never mention Windy's name . . . . Emotionally, I needed for him to talk to me. I needed to lean on him. He would hold me and let me talk, and he listened to me but never responded. This had me to the point where I was afraid to mention her name; I was holding everything in.
>
> I eventually started arguing with him about this. I knew he was very hurt by her death, and I finally realized that each person mourns the death of a child in a different way. Mine was by talking and his was by not talking. This puts a great stress on both partners, and only reasoning and compromising can help.

> Looking back with a three-year perspective, I see the holes. I thought we communicated so beautifully. But my husband didn't even begin to open himself to me about his reactions until months later. And I who talked incessantly couldn't say the things I felt most deeply until they'd been held inside so long that they simply exploded.
>
> A year later, we were still sorting through our basic reactions. My husband had not touched or held our son after he died; that had always somewhat angered me. I felt his concept that the dead body was no longer really human after the soul had gone on was too clinical in terms of one's own child. He later told me that as an only child who had not been around many infants, he couldn't remember ever having held a baby. That night he wasn't sure he wanted to fumble through learning how to hold a baby that was already dead. That I could understand.

Even the day-by-day aspects of a premature birth and an infant's hospitalization can cause problems for a couple or affect an entire family.

> This was a great strain on our family . . . . I . . . neglected [them] so badly . . . . All I could do was stay with the baby

in the hospital. I would see my little girl, [who] was staying with my mother, every other weekend for a day and
then go back to the hospital . . . . My husband and I didn't
see each other very much . . . I neglected him in many
ways as a wife . . . . To me, my baby came first.

But as time went on, I [learned] I may lose [my hus-
band] . . . . We worked things out and it couldn't be better
now. We found our love for each other was still there
. . . now there's more.

Arguments are often manifestations of the tremendous stresses
on a couple. Angry words can be an outward sign of inner frustrations and fear.

You wouldn't be normal if you didn't let off steam to the
person closest to you—each other. Remember, it can go
two ways: You can pull together or break apart. There's
much more comfort to be found in the one other person
who is as involved in the crisis as you are . . . than in your
mother, a friend or anyone else. So go ahead and fuss but
remember why you're fussing: you're tired, you're nervous and you're frightened. It does get better, believe
me.

For some couples, however, it does not get better. Extreme
crisis and undue stress have tolled the death of many a marriage.
Prematurity has led to eventual divorce for many couples.

One premature baby and 3½ years later, we are in the
process of getting a divorce. It is almost impossible to
think that our beautiful, blue-eyed little daughter could
have played any part in the circumstances that broke up
our marriage. However, my husband and I sincerely
have to agree. She did.

We had always considered our marriage a strong one.
We survived the stresses of the death of our second child.
However, the birth of our third daughter, thirteen weeks
prematurely, brought with it feelings and stress that
caused each of us to react very differently to the same
situation.

The largest single factor was the length of time we had

to endure the stress. It was two years after our daughter's delivery before we felt . . . she had outgrown most of the on-going problems of her prematurity. It was such a relief to feel that she was "normal."

Yet, after two years of giving myself so totally, and willingly, to our daughter, I was not the same [person] . . . . It's 3½ years later and our daughter is terrific. Me? All of a sudden I have my identity back. I'm not just a mother anymore. I have a growing feeling of freedom and a new sense of self-worth. There are, of course, many factors that brought [my husband and me] to where [we are] today. Our love for our daughter is total. My husband and I have absolutely no regrets about anything we did to get our 1-pound and 7-ounce baby girl to where she is today. However, the stress and circumstances surrounding her birth and the early years of her life did contribute to the breakup of our marriage.

SHARING AND SUPPORTING

Those who communicate well during the crisis of a premature birth find that their love for each other grows and their relationship is strengthened.

Sometimes, when I sat in my room and thought of all that was going on around us, I was overwhelmed . . . . The only thing that kept us sane was our love for our son and, most importantly, our love for each other.

My husband, Larry, was a tower of strength . . . . While I was still hospitalized, he would go to work in the mornings and would visit my hospital as soon as he got off and then we would visit Charlie together. He would then go home and take care of our daughter. He never stopped to do anything for himself. His fortitude was amazing.

Many couples have talked about communication problems . . . . For us, there was no lack of communication. Sometimes we didn't say a word, but we were still totally tuned into the other's thoughts and needs. Our crisis with Charlie strengthened our marriage tremendously.

There is no simple formula for establishing an open relationship. If there is any one suggestion, it is that a couple should never miss an opportunity to communicate.

> I wish I could remember all the times we had to feel our way along each other's thoughts and concerns. There were many, many things we did not understand in the ways we each reacted .... The biggest thing was learning again that we simply had to "talk it over" like all the other things we had faced before. It worked.
>
> Remarkably, I think we both were able to give each other substantial support, despite not understanding everything that was going on inside each of us. We both cared very much. Each of us knew that we were trying not to burden the other, but that in the end we each had at certain times. This was very important during the times we each were scared to death.
>
> Sharon felt somewhat guilty in regard to Susan's early birth, which was one of the things I could not understand. I thought her guilt was totally illogical, and objectively it was; but I soon learned that logic was not as important as listening and talking it over.

SOURCES OF STRESS

It is difficult for parents to be sympathetic to one another when each feels caught up on a separate emotional roller coaster ride. The ups and downs for each parent are often produced by different events. One may finally feel a ray of sunshine when the baby first grasps the parent's finger; the other may not feel a similar ray until the extent of the insurance coverage is known.

The child's welfare, financial worries, reactions to the time-consuming physical needs of the new infant, pressure or support from relatives and acquaintances and sexual tensions can cause marital stress. In addition, each individual experiences personal stress not felt by a spouse, and the couple must cope with the normal pressures of daily life.

In many instances, stress cannot be eliminated, but communication about problems can be helpful in reducing tension.

The Child's Welfare

Good communication between parents and the professionals caring for their babies is critical when questions regarding the infant's welfare are concerned. Much confusion can result if parents feel they are not being told the whole truth or if they feel that their concerns are not being taken seriously.

The ability to communicate about an infant's physical condition is bound to a knowledge and understanding of the medical problems involved. For parents, that knowledge is not always easy to obtain. It is also difficult to separate facts from emotional responses.

Two doctors may relate the same information about an infant's condition to a parent with different words and different facial and hand gestures. From those two doctors, the parent may glean two different messages and convey this confusion to others. On the other hand, how a parent acts in the nursery can be interpreted differently by different nurses. One may see the parent as high-strung; another, as overtired and concerned about the baby's welfare. Parents sometimes receive conflicting information from professionals.

> One evening, Chet felt ill and could not enter the nursery. He watched me through the window as I watched Zachary through the Isolette portholes.
>
> Outside, I saw the doctor who was doing the spinal taps on our baby stop to talk to Chet. Chet nodded and smiled at me and the baby as the doctor talked.
>
> Meanwhile, on my side of the glass, another doctor stopped to tell me that he feared Zachary was developing hydrocephalus and described the shunt they would have to put in his head. Chet told me he had watched as I had become upset, started to cry and quickly left the nursery. The doctor talking to Chet had been saying our baby was improving and that things looked good. The glass between us prevented us from hearing what the other was hearing.
>
> We received conflicting information about the milk drip machine which upset us terribly . . . . We were not sure

what to believe and were hesitant to speak up about it to the doctor or nurse, as we did not want to make anyone angry with us and affect Pauline's care.

One father, a lawyer, told of his experiences while seeking information and offered a comment:

> The staff did not harass me for chart reading while Susan was in intensive care. Frankly, heaven help them if they had! Doctors and nurses who give the intensive and critical care understand that parents can't accept not having information available. But later, in the premature nursery and at the end of a false-alarm visit to the emergency room after Susan came home, the hospital nurses told me that:
>
> a. Reading charts was a no-no.
> b. We ought not to have the information, as it might be confusing.
> c. The chart and its information is hospital property.
>
> Baloney to all three! The legal validity of the third statement is suspect, because it doesn't give the whole story. The others, for parents aching to know what's happening, are not worthy of listening to unless a parent is willing to be bulldozed.

There are some parents who never read charts. Others read charts every day. One way or the other, though, all parents want the same thing: correct and complete information about their child. A partial understanding of the child's condition can also pose a problem for the parents.

One parent may know the truth about a child's condition, but purposely not convey the total picture to a spouse.

> The day before our son was to be born, my wife's doctor told her mother and I that he didn't honestly think the baby would "stand a chance." I could not bring myself to believe what he said, nor did I tell my wife. I spent the night before his birth in my wife's room. As they took my wife to the delivery room, I reassured her everything would be all right. I silently prayed that I was right.
>
> When our son, Charlie, was finally born they told me

my wife was doing fine . . . . After about five minutes, the
nurse came back out and told me they had in a call for
radiology because he had what they called a "textbook
case of hyaline membrane." I had no idea what they
were talking about—from the window he looked fine to
me. The staff neonatologist and the head of the Neo department explained his condition to me, drew a picture
of his lungs and told me he would have to be transferred
. . . . Now I had to go to the recovery room and explain
this to my wife. Because of the anesthesia, it was almost
useless to explain. She barely knew I was there . . . . I left
her because I knew there was nothing I could do.

[At the hospital where my son was transferred], I saw
nothing but doctors, nurses, babies, machines, tubes,
hoses and wires. This was a world I had never seen before. They showed me to "Charlie's corner." There was
our son with tubes and wires everywhere. Machines
were beeping and counting, and he was gasping for
every breath he took.

What would I tell my wife? I had my own doubts as to
whether or not he would live, or what he would be like
if he did.

I returned to my wife's hospital and told her that he
was the cutest baby in the world, that I loved him and
that he would live. I did not bother to tell her that it was
I who said he would live, not the doctors.

Soon my wife was allowed to travel from her hospital
to his. She was shocked to see everything the pictures did
not show and I did not tell her.

This couple knew each other well enough so that the wife
understood what her husband had done for her. In her words, he
showed "strength." She saw his actions as courageous and protective. But every couple is different. In other relationships, where
the husband and wife do not have a similar groundwork of understanding, this type of protection can have disastrous consequences, leaving the wife, angry and shocked.

I didn't realize how serious it was until I got the bill. I
didn't know she was on the critical list. I didn't know she
was on a respirator . . . . When I got the bill, I called John

and asked him why he hadn't told me what was going on. I was angry because she could have died and I would have thought [her being on a respirator] was only precautionary. I was angry because he underestimated my emotional stability . . . . He should have known me better.

I had done a research paper on prenatal development as related to special education, and I think he thought I might overreact, knowing what could happen. [Because] I felt guilty . . . . I think . . . he was protecting me from the seriousness of the situation.

Occasionally, if the infant is born in a hospital where the staff is not open with parents, the medical knowledge a parent has may be a liability.

Financial Worries

For some, the cost of a premature birth is not a grave concern. One father said, "Money was not a problem. Our insurance covered a significant amount, and we were able to pay off the remainder." A mother commented, "Let's hear it for insurance!"

However, other parents are in a totally different position. A husband may have to take on a second job until the bills are paid. His wife may feel guilty that her husband has to shoulder the financial obligations alone or she may feel lonely and exhausted. Sometimes, the wife gets a job. Often in these instances, there is guilt or frustration in having to leave in the hands of someone else the daily care of the very child the parents have wanted so desperately to be well and at home.

Attitudes about finances sometimes change drastically.

Financial concern was one area in which my husband and I reversed roles. When the bills topped [his] annual income after the first few weeks of hospitalization, I— who am normally the more thrifty person—took the laissez-faire attitude that somehow the bills would take care of themselves, while my husband—the free spender —felt helpless and overwhelmed.

In some cases, the family's life-style is substantially altered by the continuing demand to meet financial obligations. Faced with insurmountable bills, some families are forced to declare bankruptcy, an action that may cause even more stress.

Caring for the Infant

It is not unusual for a parent to feel resentment at being neglected by a spouse who is spending countless hours caring for the baby. These feelings can begin to surface during the time the infant is hospitalized.

> After I came home from the hospital, I started a routine different from the one we had before. It was easier for me to get around since I could then drive. However, at the same time, Allen and I were sharing one car between us, so all my daily errands had to be done in the evenings. Since he worked all day and I sat at home, he was ready to reverse the schedule. He would ask if I had to go that night, or if I would stay home with him and our 2½-year-old. I rarely saw him; we were like two ships passing in the night.
>
> The stronger Shayne got, the more time I spent with her. I felt she needed the stimulation from her mother. At the same time, Allen was getting almost no attention from me because of my concern for the baby.
>
> I was burning a candle at three ends. During the day, I would take care of my older child, the afternoon was for Allen, the evening was reserved for visits to the hospital. By the time I got home around 10:30 p.m., I was physically exhausted. While all this was going on, there was no time for myself.

The negative feelings can engulf the whole family after the baby is home.

> Those first few months after Michael came home were difficult ones. He required so much attention: my nursing every four hours, his sleeping very little and so lightly that the slightest sound would cause him to cry, feedings

that continued through the night, months of colic that even medication would not completely eliminate, frequent visits to the pediatrician, frequent colds.

There didn't seem to be enough time in the day to care for him, much less for ourselves and our daughter and our home. And there was resentment. Our daughter wanted her share of attention. My husband wanted to be able to comfort Michael, but the only thing that seemed to help was nursing. And I wanted relief from the constant care, and time for myself.

We loved Michael, and we also knew we were tired and that he would outgrow his need for constant care. This knowledge helped us through those months.

Another mother looked back at her son's first months at home more than a year before and said, "I realize now that I owe my husband an apology."

There are premies who require special care at home. Infants have been sent home on monitors or oxygen or requiring respiratory therapy or other types of treatment for remaining medical problems.

Before Matt left the hospital, both my husband and I learned to care for him just as the nurses had. We learned how to care for and feed Matt via the gastrostomy, how to suction and change the tracheostomy, how to use the infant monitor. We were certified in infant CPR and we also instructed the [private duty] nurses on the night shift at home.

Matt required continuous oxygen. He experienced occasional blue spells, but the oxygen "pinked" him right up. Later he only required oxygen before, during and after a feeding. We used a room humidifier during the night.

Matt's doctor made weekly house calls throughout the summer. We didn't leave the house except for trips to the doctor or to the hospital. [One reason was that] Matt's portable oxygen tank was only good . . . for seven hours. Occasional trips to the hospital [were made] to have Matt's gastrostomy tube replaced. A slight tug would pull the tube loose.

Matt underwent subsequent procedures and had correctable eye problems. In a case like this one, the routine of child care imposed on the household severely alters the family's life-style. Adapting to such a totally different life-style can cause friction between parents.

Other Children, Relatives and Acquaintances

Relatives can put subtle pressure on a marriage during the best of times. Their support and love can be invaluable, just as their bitterness or insensitiveness can be disastrous. One man said, "Without my in-laws' love and their care for me and our daughter, this time would have been impossible for me."

One mother offered this observation concerning her parents and in-laws:

> The early days and weeks of dealing with the crisis of Bryan's prematurity were equally trying on our families as they were on us . . . . Our parents, in addition to their grave concern for the baby, also felt the stress of seeing us—their children—suffer; and they were no longer able to protect us.

In some families, grandparents unintentionally create stress.

> At the time that my twins were born, my mother was living at one end of the country with the four teens still at home . . . while my father was working at the other end of the country. I called both of them the day of the delivery.
>
> Because finances were extremely tight at the time and my father had access to a WATS line, it was arranged that he would call us every day or so and then in turn alert family and friends as to our status.
>
> Having been raised in a rather pragmatic family, I didn't question this . . . . Six weeks later, on my birthday, I found out that one of the reasons my mother had not called was because of her disappointment over my son's death. She did not call when he died; she . . . wasn't sure

that she "could be as brave as she heard I was being."

I look back now and wish things had been different. I would have liked very much to hear my mother say what I knew she was feeling.

Other children, especially young ones who cannot fully understand what is happening, can unintentionally cause stress. One four-year-old who expected twins was disappointed when her parents tried to explain that only one would come home. The grieving parents had to try to meet their own emotional needs as well as those of their daughter.

I don't quite know how we made it through those days with all the "Why this? Why that? How come? But, Mom . . ." But, like most kids, she made it better than we did.

One father recalled the reactions of various family members and his coworkers:

After Linda was resting back in her room, I called my parents. My mother was very upset—I didn't know how upset until much later. My dad tried not to let on how serious it really was.

I drove home at 6 [a.m.], and my mother-in-law was up and my next-door neighbors were there. They were all full of congratulations. They were trying to act happy for my sake, but inside I felt the joy was missing . . . . I just felt scared and tired.

At work the next day, I told everybody. People seemed afraid to say too much . . . . I felt they expected Sara to die just because of the 2-pound and 10-ounce [birthweight]. We didn't get many cards or gifts either.

Reactions of acquaintances and coworkers can be either discouraging or supportive. One husband kept a chart of his son's weight above his desk at work, and it became a center of conversation as fellow workers would come to check daily on "how Joey was getting along."

Sexual Tensions

The delicate balance between giving and receiving in a sexual relationship is often upset by the stresses that accompany a premature birth.

Fatigue, concern about the baby and, for some but not all couples, fear of another pregnancy ending in another premature birth, combine to create tension regarding sex. When this most intimate form of communication between a couple is feared or denied by one or both partners, the resulting pressure and frustration can lead to silence, angry words, tears or worse.

Extreme fatigue is, of course, detrimental to a couple's sexual relationship. While most parents of newborns eventually become tired because of a new baby's ordinary physical demands, parents of premies find themselves exhausted both physically and mentally. The internal emotional turmoil takes its toll, and the concerned parents who try to do all they can while their baby is hospitalized pay a price for their concern. However, getting adequate rest is impossible when worries about the baby or emotional outbursts intrude upon sleep.

> I told my husband there was no way! I practically "lived" at the hospital and used a breast pump seven or eight times each day as well. I was too tired to even think about making love.

For some couples, this exhaustion continues after the infant comes home, when frequent feedings combined with other needs of the baby's immature body preempt attention usually given to other things, including sex.

Underlying much of the sexual tension parents feel is the fear of another pregnancy. Many couples react strongly to a premature birth, saying that they never again want to put a child at such risk. Others approach the possibility of another pregnancy cautiously. All know that, aside from abstinence, there are no totally reliable birth-control methods. When a definite reason for the early delivery cannot be determined, the possibility of another premature birth can be haunting.

On the other hand, not all parents discount thoughts of having another child. One father, concerned about another possible premature birth, discussed some of the sexual stresses that followed the birth of his daughter and her arrival home.

> Nevertheless, there were stresses. They were, not necessarily in order: time, my wife's episiotomy, interest, preoccupation with the baby, preoccupation at times with my work and a seemingly never-ending energy crisis caused by everything that was hitting us both. To make the situation more difficult, it seemed that we were never quite "together" at the same time.

A mother who lost one prematurely born daughter visited her obstetrician while her remaining twin was still hospitalized and asked if she could become pregnant again right away.

> The doctor said that he saw no physical reason for me not to become pregnant again, but he did also say that he felt that I was not really emotionally ready for another pregnancy. In addition, my husband wasn't sure he was ready to try again.

No matter what is decided regarding future pregnancies, the stresses placed on a couple immediately after a premature birth and during a high-risk infant's first year or so of life are considerable and can greatly affect a couple's sexual relationship. For some, the idea of enjoying anything while their child is in danger seems callous and uncaring.

Unrelated Events

There are particular stresses unique to each couple because of events not directly related to the birth. A husband's business trip overseas, an older child's birthday party only days after an infant's death, the illness of a favorite aunt, even the death of a pet can cause extra tension at a time when a couple needs desperately for their world to be calm.

Two women spoke of specific stressful events surrounding the birth of their children:

My husband was about to leave the country for a three-week business trip. Although I was in a room alone during my hospital stay and I requested that he be allowed to visit, the staff emphatically refused. He could visit our baby whenever he wanted but I "needed my rest." What I needed was my husband for what little time we had. "Rest" was impossible for me.

When my husband returned, our son was just home from the hospital. We never really talked about our problems with Michael. We were so busy caring for him and his older sister that there wasn't much time left for talking. In our ten years of marriage, we had developed a nonverbal communication that saw us through those difficult first months.

Prior to [my son's] birth, I had lost my first husband, father, grandmother and grandfather. The greatest tragedy of my life was happening at the same time: My mother was dying of cancer. She was living with me . . . [while] getting treatment. She fought hard to hold on since our child was her only grandchild—a new inspiration for living. She died four months after his birth. (She saw very little of him because of her illness and his.)

So possibly my child's hospitalization wasn't as devastating as to others for whom this is their first meeting with tragedy. To me, there is no comparison between the death of a newborn and someone [with whom] you have shared years of love. Yet each is a great loss.

[When] I had a miscarriage [at three months] this past summer . . . . it was a blow, but I kept it all in proper perspective. We just hope another day will bring us a healthy, full-term child.

HOSPITAL RECORDS

The ownership and control of hospital records can be a problem when parents seek information about their child's medical condition. While some hospitals prohibit parents from reading charts, others have less stringent rules.

In seeking information, parents should know, first of all, that "the ownership of medical records rests with the hospital, or with the physician who keeps records of private patients in his office." (ArthurF.Southwick, *The Law of Hospital and Health Care Administration*) Such records include daily charts, X rays and other laboratory reports, nurses' notes and similar documents. The right to physical possession rests with the owner of the records (that is, with the hospital or the doctor).

However, this does not mean that parents can be summarily denied access to medical records and the information in them. The guideline for access is that the person must have a legitimate reason to see the record and "must comply with reasonable safeguards established by the physician or hospital to assure the physical safety of the record while inspection is taking place." (The Law of Hospital and Health Care.)

In their book, *The Rights of Parents,* attorneys Alan N. Sussman and Martin Guggenheim discuss the rights of parents to be informed about medical treatment given to their children. While the answer is unclear in the case of adolescents, because of the doctrine of "privileged" communication between doctor and patient, Sussman and Guggenheim note that "when a patient is an infant or a small child, there is no question that the 'privilege' between doctor and patient includes the parent."

"If a parent takes a child to a doctor for treatment and the child is quite young, the answer is that the parent has a right to be told virtually everything. Parents are charged with providing adequate medical care for their children. They must also pay for the medical services their children receive. Therefore, they have a right to know what type of treatment and care their children are given. This includes the severity of the malady, the type of medication and all other relevant aspects of a child's medical or hospital care."

Thus, while parents do not have an unlimited opportunity to personally study medical records, they do have the right to the information in them and in many cases some reasonable access to the records themselves.

Chapter 6

BUT IT'S OUR BABY!

During pregnancy, mothers and fathers fantasize not only about the baby's sex and appearance but also about the baby's arrival. Plans are made based on a calculated due date. Parents may anticipate labor as difficult and tiring work, but they usually expect birth itself to be a joyous event, a cause for celebration. When a baby is born prematurely, the celebration is postponed; concern replaces the expected happiness.

The subsequent hospitalization and the separation of babies from their mothers and fathers violates the expectations of parents and the norms of society.

Before our son's birth, a neighbor brought home her newborn son. Neighbors, myself included, flocked to see the baby. This is normal in our society. New babies are almost public property. Parents proudly show off their newborn, and friends and relatives come to celebrate.

The interesting comment made by this neighbor was that in cattle, when a new calf is born, the rest of the herd will gather around and inspect the new member. In this way, the calf is recognized and accepted as part of the herd. In many ways, this is true of our human society also.

So what happens when a baby is born prematurely or is ill . . . and is separated from the parents and their families and friends for long periods of time? . . . When the baby finally comes home, parents are constantly reminded by others and by their restricted life-style that their baby is not like "normal" newborn babies. Basically, the "herd," or society, has missed its opportunity to inspect the new member.

This quote is from a woman who has experienced three troubled pregnancies. She further observed:

My best explanation of the "missing something" in my relationship with my son is my lack of relaxation into "normal" motherhood during his first year. I believe most new mothers lose their fear of their babies' fragility after caring for them the first few weeks of life. A premature baby's hospitalization and the . . . isolation of the baby and parents that sometimes follows doesn't allow the new family to relax into a regular routine.

Her words touch on several aspects of separation: the absence of celebration, the lack of societal approval, the tension of the situation and, above all, the abnormality of the birth.

In one way or another, parents attempt to adjust to this abnormal atmosphere both during their child's hospitalization and afterwards. They express concern about their babies' difficult beginnings, they try to cope with the surrealism of this "absentee" parenthood, they rebel, they protest, they feel cheated, they try to equalize the forces that seem to be working against them (that is, the hospital regulations and their children's illnesses). Most parents eventually cope with the experience in their own ways.

The separation of parents and their babies can be divided into four main categories: initial separation after birth, transfer babies who are sent to other hospitals, a prolonged hospital stay for the infant and second-time separations, where a child must be readmitted to the hospital after having come home.

INITIAL SEPARATION

We had gone through so much the past seven months. We had given up hope of having a baby, so separation should not be hard. Yet, as I lay in my hospital room and listened to a baby's cry from the next room, I missed mine. I felt hurt that I could not hold Sara in my arms and kiss her. I felt I was missing out on something that would never be offered to me again.

Due to this mother's near death from the complications of toxemia, she eventually had a tubal ligation and will, in fact, never again have the chance to hold her own baby soon after birth. Because of the seriousness of their conditions, Sara and her mother would probably have been separated in any hospital in this country. Nothing, however, can totally erase the disappointment the mother felt.

Because of a premature birth, parents may not see their baby immediately after delivery. Many of those who do see the baby at birth recall having a positive, and often optimistic, feeling. On the other hand, some parents, stunned by the baby's small size and appearance, fear that such a tiny, fragile infant cannot possibly survive.

Many who do not have the opportunity to see their newborn baby feel they have missed out on an important event.

> I wish now that I could have seen him. I realize that I was groggy, but the staff nurses never asked if I wanted a look. It might not have had a big impact on me at the time, since I was rather sleepy, but now I wish I had those moments to remember.
>
> My husband said his first thought was of how beautiful Joey looked. Joey was breathing rapidly and it was an apparent struggle for him to breathe, but Joe loved him. I guess that everyone was trying to protect me from an unpleasant experience. Instead I feel I missed out on something beautiful.

For some mothers, feeding time at the hospital is especially difficult. They know their babies will not be coming.

I resented having a roommate who was able to receive her baby at feeding time. Gr-r-r. It made me so mad; I was so envious. I knew this was probably the only child I would ever give birth to; why couldn't it be right?

I hated the ignorant nurses who would ask, "Don't you want to feed your baby, Mrs. Kauffman?" Why couldn't they take the time to find out that my baby was not able to come to me before awakening me at 2 a.m. for a feeding? Why did I have to inform them, "You won't find him on this floor. He is in NICU"?

Visiting the Nursery

Even when allowed to visit, touch or hold their baby, parents feel the stress of trying to be a family in the nursery. There is usually little privacy there, and the physical aspects of the medical care make it difficult to cuddle and caress a baby the way most parents do with their healthy newborns. Wires and IVs are not conducive to close physical contact. If the baby is on oxygen and in an incubator, parents may only be allowed to open the portholes for a few minutes at a time. A parent may even be excluded from the nursery because of infections, colds or contagious illnesses.

While most concerned parents respect the rules needed to protect their children, many also rebel against what they consider excessive regulations.

Nonetheless, the act of holding their own child is a necessity for most parents, no matter what the restrictions. It is an event they dream of beforehand and relive afterward.

My husband and I both got to hold Ryan for the first time at eleven days of age. His nurse bundled him, his tubes and wires with ease. I sat holding Ryan, my husband holding the oxygen tube, the two of us enmeshed in the tubes and wires that connected our baby to his life-support systems.

I didn't get to hold him again until he was seven weeks old. I finally got up my nerve and went to his doctor and told him I needed to become more involved with my child. We sat down and had quite a chat. From the next day on, I was allowed to hold him and then was given more and more responsibility for daily chores . . . . I loved it . . . . I thrived on it.

Sara's mom said, "Many times I had to grit my teeth [to keep] from crying out, 'Let me hold my baby.' " Mindy's mother, who lost one of her twins and did not hold her surviving daughter until a nurse asked if she wanted to, told this story:

> I was so excited, but I really was scared to death. She weighed 1 pound and 9 ounces at the time, and she still was on CPAP. I held her, kissed her on the forehead and told her that I loved her. Her heart rate started dropping so I handed her to the nurse quickly. It was three more weeks before I got to sit back and enjoy holding my little 2-pound baby.

For many parents, the initial absence of eye contact with their baby is a significant disappointment.

> More than being physically separated, we were separated from the new-baby rituals that nature has developed. For example, mothers and fathers are denied their opportunity to inspect their baby privately, to recognize its features and, I think, to accept it as their own child.
>
> One of the most painful losses for me was not seeing Zachary's eyes opened until nearly two weeks had passed. There was a real need in me to look into my son's eyes.

Leaving the hospital is always difficult. Sara's father recalled:

> It was very difficult to leave. I'd always stand outside the nursery window after she was back in the incubator, and I never remember leaving without praying for her—that made it easier to leave. I always felt kind of lonesome walking out of the hospital by myself.

Some mothers even admit to thoughts of stealing their babies from the hospital.

One time I couldn't get up to see her during the day. So
I went at night, which was a mistake. All I wanted to do
was grab her and run—anywhere, so long as I got her out
of there.

Occasionally, a well-meaning obstetrician or other concerned
person will attempt to prevent a mother from visiting the nursery "for her own good."

Ryan's mother countermanded her obstetrician's orders to stay
away from her son after the neonatologists caring for him admitted that there was no real reason for her not to see him:

I knew Ryan was very sick, but when I looked down at
him, the enormous, miraculous machines with their in-
cessant noise shrank very much into the background. He
was my son . . . how very fantastic. He was the miracle.
His arms were taped down but his fingers were free
. . . . I caressed them. It was only for a few minutes, but
enough physical contact to last me for hours. How we
needed each other! Now I could go back upstairs and
have something to hang on to.
Just seeing him gave me such a lift. I guess that [can be]
something very difficult for a male obstetrician to understand, . . . the strength and importance of the maternal
instinct.

Nursery visitations can provide poignant moments that border
on parody.

I had held a dead child, and I wasn't offered the chance
to hold his sister for 3½ weeks. I was practically eu-
phoric, rocking my pink-blanketed bundle . . . but all my
husband seemed to be concerned with was keeping
enough slack on the IV tube, not letting our daughter get
cold . . . . I had to tell him in no uncertain terms to back
off! I was going to hold my baby with him or without him.

Separation for Parents With Older Children

Although a baby's hospitalization can be trying for any family,
parents who have already cared for full-term infants may find the

circumstances even more difficult to accept. Their expectations are based on prior experiences. Comparisons are almost inevitable. It can be even more difficult to deal with the physical aspects of caring for children at home during a time of such crises or with the emotional aspects of coping with an older child's perceptions of the infant's hospitalization.

> Coming home to an expectant almost-two-year-old without the new baby was painful. We still felt tender from the sudden early arrival and our daughter could sense our concern.
>
> We admitted this concern to her rather than lie and say that everything was fine—which it wasn't. We tried to answer her questions fully without getting too lengthy or involved in our explanations.
>
> We took her with us to shop for the baby and encouraged her to help prepare the room for her new brother at home. But we tried not to overdo any of this. There was quite enough traveling to and from the hospital to visit baby without a lot of extras.

On the other hand, one mother commented that having an older child at home made the separation a little easier:

> Of course, a two-year-old is demanding, but that kept my mind occupied .... His excitement and enthusiasm about his baby brother kept me thinking about the day Ryan would come home and what a happy twosome they would make. He kept my heart light when it was so very easy to get down and discouraged.

TRANSFER BABIES

It is usually a great shock for the parents if their baby is transferred to a larger, better-equipped hospital. The feeling of loss is often intense for the mother, who may have not yet been able to have any contact with her baby. Both parents may be chilled by the knowledge that their child is so ill as to require transfer. In fact, the baby may not be desperately ill; a cautious pediatrician or neonatologist may simply want the baby to be at the hospital with the best facilities. In any case, a transfer intensifies the separation between parents and children.

> It was like they were taking part of me away . . . . When I walked in the halls, I always ended up at the nursery. I would stand back and watch all the happy couples making happy faces at their babies through the glass. I watched new parents with friends and relatives laughing and showing off their new little "bundles of joy."
>
> My "bundle of joy" was at another hospital gasping for every breath he took. I was glad that these people did not have to know the pain and sadness we were feeling, but at the same time I was jealous of their carefree life.
>
> I think the entire experience would have been easier in the beginning if Charlie and I could have been in the same hospital. At least I would have been able to be with him more and could have seen him anytime I was having doubts about him.

To lessen a mother's feeling of loss when a baby is transferred, some hospital nurseries use instant-print cameras to take photographs of the baby prior to or immediately after transfer. Some fathers may buy or borrow instant-print cameras so they can photograph the baby themselves and take prints to anxiously waiting mothers. Mothers usually cling to these photographs in the days they are separated from their babies.

In some situations, a woman can request that her obstetrician give her a pass to leave the hospital of birth and go to the transfer hospital to visit the baby. Her request may be honored if she is physically able to travel.

A transfer is difficult for fathers, too, who spend precious time and energy traveling between the two hospitals.

In many units, the baby's nurses are available twenty-four hours a day to talk to parents on the telephone. Some hospitals even maintain toll-free numbers for parents who live far from the hospital.

A transfer hospital is usually farther from the baby's home, making visitation more difficult.

After a two-week stay at the hospital, I could feel the effects of separation—not only was I able to see Karen only once a day for short periods, but traveling the long distance was getting difficult. When she was transferred back to the local hospital, I could visit quite often and for longer periods of time, which eased the separation. In fact, it was almost as if she had come home once she was transferred closer to us. In reality, though, I viewed it as one step closer to home.

Some parents travel long distances, 100 miles or more, to visit their children. In such cases, daily visits are an impossibility. Later transfers bring different frustrations.

Having been teased by the nurses at one hospital about our preparations for Trey's homecoming, the transfer orders hit particularly hard. It had been two months of struggle for Trey. We had thought things were headed in the right direction. His blood pressure just didn't cooperate with our hopes and dreams.

Our ride to the other hospital that night seemed more dreadful than the one two months earlier when, bleeding and scared but still pregnant, I arrived at the hospital where Trey was born.

Hospital staffs can do much to ease the strain on parents. Ryan was transferred twice.

Both hospitals made us feel very welcome and involved with our baby. By the time Ryan was transferred to his last hospital, which was to make visitations easier for us, the nurses had passed the word ahead . . . that we were doing many of the daily chores . . . . for our child.

This made our last hospital stay much more pleasant. The nurses trusted that we were capable and they pretty much left us alone, which was great.

When Ryan was transferred to this last hospital—from a large children's hospital to a smaller community hospital —he was found to have a minute fungal growth and he was considered "contaminated."

That sounds bad, but it really was not. What it meant was that Ryan was isolated from the rest of the babies in the nursery.

At first I thought, "Oh, no. No more isolation for this little boy. He's had enough of that by being in an Isolette for 2½ months." But the results were nice. He was in a room by himself, which allowed us much privacy.

PROLONGED HOSPITAL STAYS

At the onset of premature labor, parents are often forewarned about possible consequences of early birth. Generally, neonatologists suggest that parents be prepared for a hospital stay lasting approximately until the baby's projected due date. However, some infants are released well before their due date, while others are hospitalized much longer. The length of the hospital stay depends upon the infant's medical condition.

Even when parents have an idea of what to expect, questions remain. At the start of her labor, one mother went through this chain of thought:

> When I learned that my labor could not be postponed for any significant time, I began remembering the stories my mother had told me about her own experience when I was born four to six weeks early almost thirty years ago.
>
> She had not been allowed in the nursery for the six weeks I stayed in the hospital and had not been awake when I was born. She had told me many times how difficult it had been for her.
>
> I felt better knowing that I would at least get to see my baby because my obstetrician planned on giving me an epidural [anesthesia] for delivery, but I had no idea how the hospital nursery now handled situations regarding premature babies and their parents.

Bonding

The topic of maternal-infant bonding has received much attention in recent years. Popular magazines have featured articles on this concept, claiming that there is a sensitive period immediately after birth during which mothers most easily develop an emotional attachment to their babies.

Bonding often becomes an intense issue for those who have read about it, either in articles or in the literature of Dr. Marshall H. Klaus and Dr. John H. Kennell. These two American doctors brought the matter of bonding to the attention of the medical community, and in doing so, they helped open the doors of special care nurseries to parents.

Some parents familiar with this concept fear that the lack of interaction with their infants at birth and subsequent loss of intimacy during the hospitalization may have long-range detrimental effects on their ability to parent. Others are concerned that separation might interfere with the child's ability to bond with them.

> I must admit, I did get a little obsessed with . . . bonding. I was never afraid that I wouldn't be attached to my baby, but instead that his three-month hospital stay would leave him a cold, unresponsive little boy. But he was so special to us, [so] that's the way we treated him and [now] it shows. Today, sixteen months later, he is a warm, loving, happy baby.

> While I was pumping milk for the umpteenth time, . . . I wondered silently, "Susan, I'm working so hard to bond with you. I sit here with this breast pump day after day. I go to the hospital every day to bathe, feed, diaper and hold you, even when I am tired. I worry about you. But are you in any way bonding with me?"

Other parents reject the notion that separation means that bonding with their baby will be significantly delayed or never occur.

> I knew nothing about the term "bonding" at Karen's birth . . . After I discovered this term, I realized that I had found [my own] ways to bond with my baby. I brought breast milk to her, dressed her and brought toys. The only physical benefit she received was the milk; the rest was for us—the parents. We were doing things for her as

though she were home. We felt we had "bonded" to our baby.

Then I heard a speaker talking about child abuse by parents of premature infants and wondered if perhaps that was down the road somewhere for us. No, that just didn't make sense.

Since I had never read anything about maternal-infant bonding and the effects of separation, I didn't dwell on any problems that could have arisen from it. All I knew was that I loved my baby no matter where she was and no "theory" could ever prove that there might not be a bond between us.

Whether or not parents are concerned with bonding as an issue, most are greatly affected by the separation and its effects.

[The] separation was quite difficult. Mothers are not made to have babies and leave them, no matter how good the reason or the place caring for the baby.

Parents may not realize that research on bonding was partially a result of experiences with premature infants and their mothers. When mothers were prohibited from being in the nurseries, doctors noted, as did early neonatologist Dr. Pierre C. Budin, that some mothers later showed little or no interest in their babies. When mothers were permitted in the nurseries, better maternal-child relations were often observed. Recent research indicates that, although contact during this bonding period can be important, the impact of separation at birth can be overcome.

In truth, deep attachments develop over time. Through special efforts by parents with the support and encouragement of the medical professionals, bonding of parents and their infant can be fostered even in the hospital setting.

Barriers

Although the nursery may be the perfect environment for the ill newborn, it often forms a physical barrier between parents and their infants. Parents often linger at the nursery window before leaving just to spend a few extra minutes looking at their child. One mother commented on an unusual aspect of those moments:

> Many times, we would be the ones outside the window staring in, waiting for the visiting hour. Then we were trapped into hearing the comments of people passing in the hall.
>
> Some stopped to gawk at the tiny babies. Some would very knowingly tell a companion that "all those babies couldn't possibly live." Or they would discuss how painful the IVs and monitors looked on the "poor little things," and then be thankful it hadn't been their own child. Some would talk to us, commenting on the antics of the babies, jerking on gavage tubes and monitor wires or inching their way into the corners of the Isolettes.
>
> I often felt compelled to let them know quickly that our son was in the nursery. Even though it subjected us to many questions, I felt it saved some poor unsuspecting gawker from "informing" us of our son's chances for survival and then having to deal with my emotional outburst.

Inside the nursery, parents feel barred from contact with their infant by the incubators, oxygen hoods and other medical equipment.

In addition to physical barriers, parents sense the unseen barriers that result from various hospital policies like the necessity to scrub before entering the nursery.

> It was like your mother saying for the third time, "They are not clean yet; go and wash them again and this time, I want them clean."
>
> Before we ever left the house, we scrubbed ourselves like you do for your first date. We avoided contact with anything other than items necessary to get to the hospital. Then after passing the windowed wall of the nursery and seeing Trey kicking (probably angry about our late arrival!), we went through the last barrier between us and our son, scrubbing and gowning. Betabutalin, the same as used by surgeons, up to the elbow, lather good,

rinse, now no touching. We would assist one another into gowns . . . . I felt like Dr. Kildare beside Ben Casey.

I would grab my purse out of habit. "Oh, well, go on George. I'll wash again and be right in."

I often wondered if Trey could in fact "feel my presence" through all those layers.

Even in hospitals that allow parents to care for their children in limited ways, parents may seldom or never have a chance to bathe their infants. Mothers have been known to say that a special nurse "secretly" permitted them to change their babies' diapers.

Medical complications can result in a child receiving specialized care that may prevent parental involvement. For example, a baby's diapers may need to be weighed before and after changing to monitor exactly how much is eliminated in comparison to the intake of fluids. The nursery staff can either prohibit parents from diapering this child, since special attention is necessary, or they can show parents where the scale is kept so that the parents can change the infant and weigh the soiled diaper themselves.

Another common example is the case of a baby with continuing respiratory problems. Such a baby may need a daily regimen of respiratory therapy or chest postural drainage, commonly called "cupping and clapping," to break up and dislodge mucus in the lungs. A child may be well enough to be discharged but require treatments at home. Parents who have not been taught how to do the therapy may be uncomfortable assuming the responsibility for such "nursing" care at home.

Hospital policies that prohibit or severely limit parental involvement are the result of many factors. The medical staff may believe that the nursery must be kept as sterile as possible, or the hospital administration may fear lawsuits by parents. These factors may cause the hospital to take a cautious view of the changes needed to eliminate restrictive policies.

"Does My Baby Recognize Me?"

Many parents wonder, "Does my baby know me?" Some medical experts believe that premature infants are incapable of recognizing their parents at birth and shortly thereafter because of their immaturity. Other experts, and a good many parents, disagree.

Actually, the real question may be whether parents can recognize their baby. Finding their baby's incubator moved to a new position in the nursery panics some parents who fear they might not know which baby is theirs. Parents may wonder, too, if their infant can differentiate them from among the many nurses and doctors who are around the baby so constantly.

Whatever the reality, parents have a strong sense of being cheated. On the day Zachary was expected to leave the hospital, his mother wrote in her journal:

> Wishing doesn't make it so. Hoping makes it harder. You're not home yet. Today, I thought you'd be here with me. Wrong. Wrong. I hurt so. Yes, I cry for myself. I sit in your empty room. I tell your yellow bear how beautiful you are—how much I want you home. I cry and get angry when people tell me it will be soon. "Soon" has been for the past six weeks.
>
> I can't sleep well at night. I don't want to talk to anyone. I'm tired of talking and schedules and hospitals and rules. You know me less than you know the nurses. I saw that last night. The nurse held you and talked to you, and you watched her the way you watched me. I'm no different. You don't know your mother. I have no spare emotions.

Often, the simple observation by a nurse or another person indicating that a baby does indeed respond to his or her parents is reassuring. Parents may be too preoccupied and tense to notice their infant's responsiveness for themselves.

> In a conversation with Susan's nurses one evening, I commented that it seemed as though she woke up just as we arrived every evening.
>
> One of the nurses replied that she too had noticed this and that many babies do become accustomed to their parents' visiting patterns.
>
> Then she recalled with a smile one baby whose father

was a security guard at the medical center. His shift ended at 2 a.m., and every morning, he would come to the nursery after work to play with his baby.

"That baby usually woke up just before or right as the father arrived," said the nurse. Shaking her head, she added, "I can just imagine the problems those parents had getting that baby to adjust to sleeping at night!"

SUBSEQUENT SEPARATION

Parents who have had some idea of what to expect from a hospital experience can find readmission to the hospital more difficult to handle than the initial separation.

Some parents whose children return to the hospital frequently find that emotional support from other parents with similar experiences is helpful in coping with the frustration and worry that accompany each hospital admission. One organization that encourages and promotes open, flexible visiting policies for parents with hospitalized children is Children in Hospitals, Inc., 31 Wilshire Park, Needham, Massachusetts 02192.

> Two weeks after Karen came home from the hospital, she became ill with viral pneumonia and was hospitalized for another ten days. This time I really felt as though my child was being taken from me—not by the hospital, but by the illness. There we were again, driving back downtown to visit our daughter who had become so much a part of our family. She would be handled once more by strangers.

Some babies have long-range problems that require frequent rehospitalization. The frustrations and expense involved can be staggering. On the other hand, a mother whose son had numerous medical difficulties and was hospitalized after his homecoming for eye surgery and suturing of the opening left by his tracheostomy had a different view:

> Matt's hospitalizations were for reasons that were not life-threatening . . . . We knew they would take place

. . . but we looked on these visits to the hospital in a good light because they were a sign of his getting better. There was always the worry of a child being hospitalized . . . but there was always the good feeling that he'd be coming home on one less piece of equipment.

MAKING THE SEPARATION EASIER

There are a number of things a parent can do to make the separation less difficult. In addition to asking to become involved in their infant's daily care, they should also remember that playing with their baby is important.

However, parents should be alert to any signs of overstimulation. Too many activities, too many stimuli, may be overwhelming, especially to very early premies.

Some parents find that keeping a journal provides an outlet for their emotions and a written record for the future. Others collect mementos for a baby book—a lock of hair, for instance—or take photographs documenting the baby's progress.

Some mothers busy themselves sewing tiny hospital gowns, if clothing is permitted in the nursery. Parents may search stores for small-size clothes or tiny toys. Other mothers faithfully use a breast pump to provide milk for their baby. Fathers can take milk to the hospital and offer encouragement.

Most parents find that staying busy helps keep up their spirits and minimize their fear.

Here are a few guidelines on coping with separation:

1. Relax. Parents preoccupied with every wire and monitor are probably missing some special moments with their child. It is true that parents need to know what is being done for their baby, but medical care should be left to the medical professionals. Parents should make every attempt to make the most of the time they have with their child. Body language is an important form of communication.

2. Trust that an attachment between parents and child will grow. Even before babies open their eyes, smile,

or grasp their mothers' or fathers' fingers, they sense their love. Attachments can be developed over time if the child feels love.

3. Learn not to be discouraged. Even if there is no room where parents and their child can be alone or if a child is too sick to be taken from the incubator or warmer, parents can communicate with their baby even if it is limited to hand-holding through the portholes of an incubator.

4. Work with the hospital staff when you honestly feel changes can be made. Parents who feel capable of assuming some of the baby's daily care should ask to do so. Most hospitals are willing at least to consider suggestions for improvement.

5. Take one day at a time. It is a good idea to resolve concerns on a daily basis. Medical questions, in particular, should be asked and answered as quickly as possible. It is wise for parents to deal with the facts related to their baby's condition and to try not to be overwhelmed by negative possibilities.

"DO YOU EVER GET OVER IT?"

This question is asked hundreds of times. Sometimes parents think they are "over it"; then the memory of a shaved head, a childhood illness or a nightmare about the child dying jars them to the realization that the separation really did occur.

Parents need not try to "get over it" by pushing the experience aside. Instead, they should try to put what was learned into proper perspective.

> Those first few days of Susan's life when she was fighting to survive were frightening to me, but they also touched something deep in my soul. There are times when I stand in absolute awe of the determination my daughter showed in claiming her right to live.
>
> The pain of our separation will never be forgotten, but I hope that instead of a lasting scar it has made me aware of just how precious our time together is.

First Visit

I was led to our reunion
an early child and mother.
Our bracelets matched;
assurance of belonging
to one another.

You lay naked in a false tropic;
a greenhouse orchid of rare pallor.
Touch could bruise your translucence.
The curled leaf of an ear defied secrets
once ours . . .

The room pulsed of droning bees and
exotic, mechanical birdsong;
I was dizzy in the heat.

Threats of tears and screaming milk
were gathering like the mist
that was a shroud about your face.
I yearned to see your eyes
or have my finger caught
in your hands' embrace.

I was led from our reunion,
a fragile child and mother.
Our spirits matched;
assurance of belonging
to one another.

Sherry Pearson

PREMIE PLAYTIME*

Premature babies, like other infants, need stimulation of all their senses, both during their hospital stay and after they come home. Because many of a premie's first experiences in the world are negative ones (having blood drawn, being intubated, etc.), it is important for their future development that gentle and loving stimulation also be provided.

From the very start, you can encourage your baby to feel like a member of the family. Touch your baby; if allowed, hold your baby; make all the sweet, cooing sounds you would if you were in the privacy of your own home. While touching or stroking, talk to your child. Call your baby by name, ask how he or she is doing, talk about your thoughts. Don't forget to smile at your baby! Your presence, voice, touch, scent, warmth and feelings of love are important and will be communicated by your actions.

VISUAL STIMULATION.   Most appealing to newborns are vivid contrasts and repetitious patterns, such as a bull's eye or checkerboard. Babies also respond to the human face; show your baby the "Pampers" baby on the diaper box. Any design, mobile, etc., should be placed on one side of the baby's bed, since at this early age, babies keep their heads turned to one side or the other.

AUDITORY STIMULATION.   Talk to your baby! Sing! Play a music box for him, or wind up a stuffed musical toy. If you provide a recorder, ask the nurses to play a cassette tape of soothing music or voices of family members. When recording, family members may read a nursery rhyme or poem, sing, talk to the baby or just say "I love you."

TACTILE STIMULATION.   Touch your baby whenever possible, even if it must be through the portholes of an incubator. Gently massage, stroke, handle, cuddle and rock your baby. Ask the nursery staff to let you give your baby his daily bath. Afterwards, your infant may enjoy an oil rub . . . an excellent time for touching and massaging.

Every baby has an alert state; ask the nursery staff to help you identify this period. Take advantage of this time to touch, hold, talk to, sing to and play with your baby.

A word of caution: A premature baby needs lots of rest. Overstimulation can be as harmful as a lack of appropriate stimulation.

Watch for signs of overstimulation—grimacing, excessive crying, turning away.

The nursing staff and your doctor can guide you in stimulating your baby's senses.

*Adapted from "Premie Playtime" by Parents of Prematures, Houston.

PERSONALIZING YOUR BABY*

Most hospitals now permit (and some even encourage) parents to get acquainted with their new baby as soon as possible and to "personalize" the baby. Giving your son or daughter his or her own identity can make the stay at the hospital a bit less difficult.

1. Put pictures of family members on the incubator, or spell out your baby's name with colorful, bold letters.
2. Record the voices of baby's mother, father, grandparents, brothers and sisters on a cassette. Place a recorder in the incubator and ask nurses to play it periodically so that your baby will recognize the voices when he comes home.
3. Buy or make toys for your baby. Keep the size of the incubator in mind; select small, safe toys that will not interfere with equipment. Remember that toys must withstand the heat and moisture of the incubator. Music boxes and musical stuffed toys are a soothing alternative to the unending monotonous beep . . . beep . . . beep of the monitors.
4. Decorate a box or bag for your baby's belongings— extra booties, caps, toys. Personalize the container: "Michael's Miscellaneous," "Julie's Junk," etc.
5. Buy or sew clothes for your baby. Booties and caps are often the first items a baby is permitted to wear in the nursery. Stocking-type booties stay on best, and caps that fit can usually be found, since a premie's head size is usually not much smaller than a term baby's. Most nurseries discourage caps that tie under the chin. Clothes should be loose, simple and comfortable. Kimonos or gowns allow doctors and

nurses easy access to your baby; save "dressy" outfits for your baby's homecoming, visits to the pediatrician and other special occasions. Keep in mind that all garments should keep baby comfortably warm, be soft and smooth and be easy to launder.

Because hospital policies vary greatly, check with your doctor and the nursing staff before following any of these suggestions.

*Adapted from "Personalizing Your Baby" by Parents of Prematures, Houston.

Chapter 7

HOMECOMING AND FIRST YEARS

We knew that if all went well Monica would be home on Monday. The Friday before, I called the nursery from work to check on her progress, and the nurse who answered told me that I could take her home that day. I put the nurse on hold and shouted the news to the people around me . . . . Daryel and I agreed to pick her up at the earliest time possible, which was nine o'clock that evening.

Then it all hit me. Nothing was ready . . . . I didn't even have diapers or formula at home.

I called my ever-faithful friend, Margaret, who came over and took me to the store. (At that time, I had not yet learned to drive.) She told me her sister could lend me a bassinet until her own baby was born. Then she steered me to the diapers . . . suddenly we realized I didn't even have a diaper pail!

As I stood in line to pay for my purchases, I laughed and cried out loud. I know everyone must have wondered about me, but that didn't matter . . . . Monica was really alive, and she was really coming home.

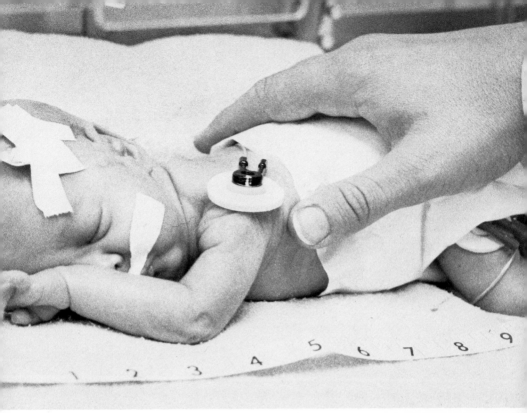

Figure 1. While size is not the only criterion of prematurity, most early babies weigh less than 5½ pounds. This baby, for example, is small enough to fit into her father's hand.
Photo by Sherri Nance.

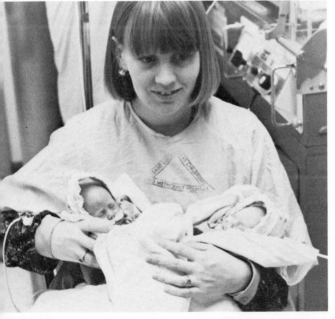

Figure 2. Multiple births are frequently premature. Marilyn holds her twin daughters, Johanna (l) and Suzanne (r), who arrived twelve weeks early. Each weighed slightly more than two pounds at birth.
Photo by Harry Bick.

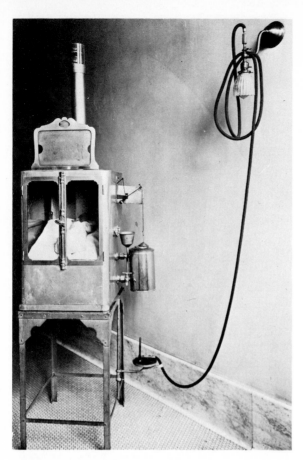

Figure 3. Early glass-walled incubators like the one shown in this 1899 photograph taken in the Sloane Maternity Center in New York allowed mothers and fathers to see their premature babies.
Photo courtesy of Byron, The Byron Collection, Museum of the City of New York.

Figure 4. Timely transport is critical for premies who need the specialized care available in an NICU. This Life Flight team from Hermann Hospital in Houston, Texas, has transferred hundreds of premature babies from outlying community hospitals to Hermann's Turner Neonatal Intensive Care Unit.
Photo by Craig Stotts.

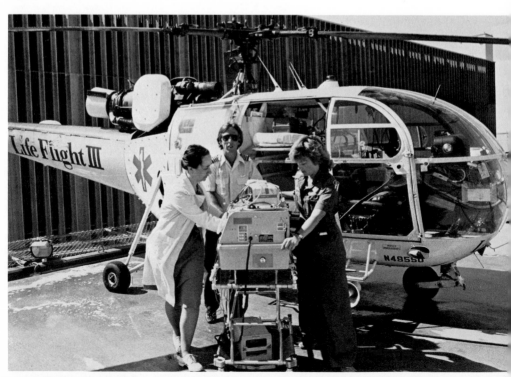

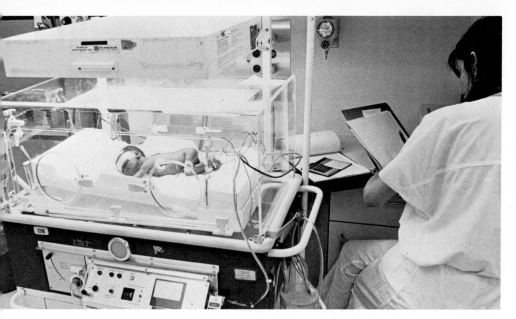

Figure 5. Phototherapy is used to treat jaundice. This premie, with eyes
blindfolded for protection, sleeps under the "bili" lights while the nurse
checks her patient's chart.
Photo by: Craig Stotts.

Figure 6. Acute respiratory distress prompts quick action in the NICU.
The head nurse listens to the heartbeat while doctors prepare to give a
blood transfusion to this newborn. An oxygen hood covering the baby's
head delivers additional oxygen to the infant to ease his labored
breathing.
Photo by Charlotte Brooks, Magnum Photos.

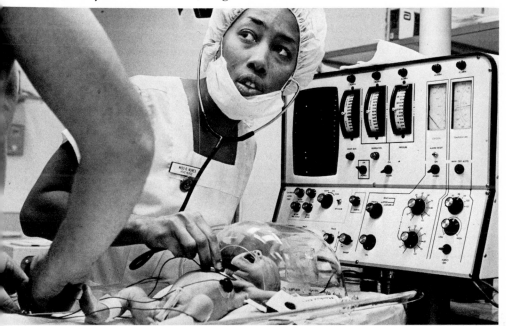

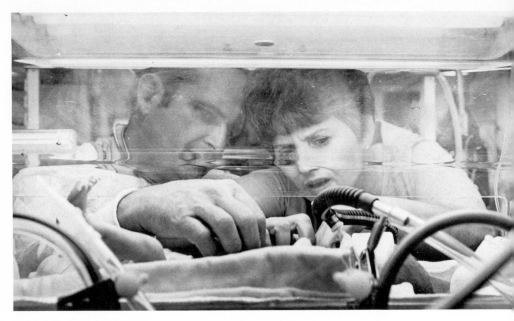

Figure 7. Anxious faces reveal these parents' concern for their new baby. Some of the anxiety that parents often feel can be eliminated or reduced by a better understanding of the equipment and procedures used in special care nurseries.
Photo courtesy of March of Dimes National Foundation.

Figure 8. That first visit to the nursery is usually an intense, unforgettable experience. These parents keep watchful eyes on their newborn daughter, as the baby's father gently strokes his daughter's tiny foot.
Photo by Craig Stotts.

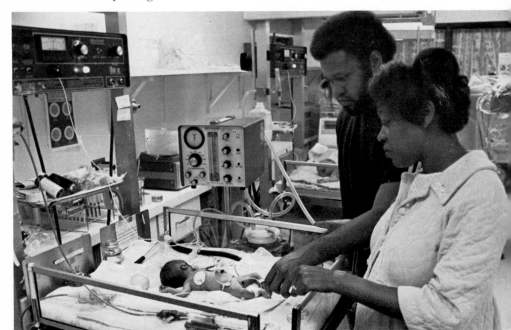

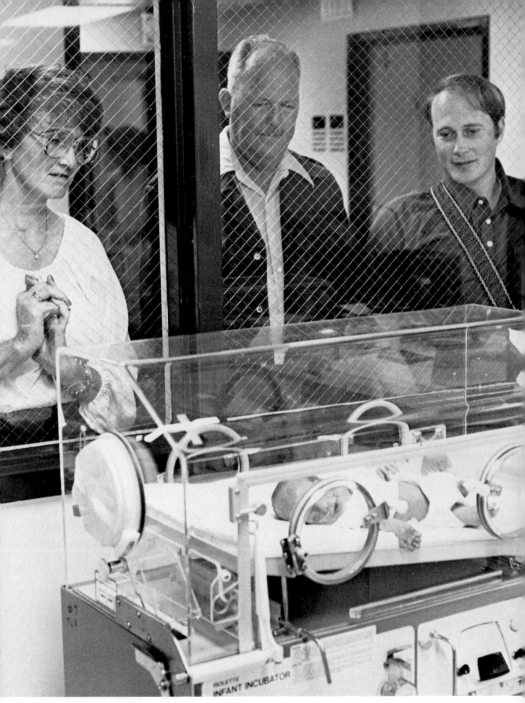
Figure 9. Premature birth causes stress for all members of a family, including new grandparents, who often must wait outside the nursery. In addition to concern for their new grandchild, many feel an added burden of seeing their own children, the baby's parents, subjected to the strain of having a baby in the hospital.

Photo by Craig Stotts.

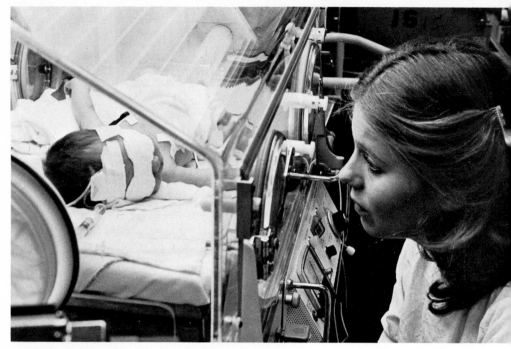

Figure 10. This mother watches her child undergoing phototherapy. Many parents miss having eye contact with their newborns. Photo courtesy of March of Dimes National Foundation.

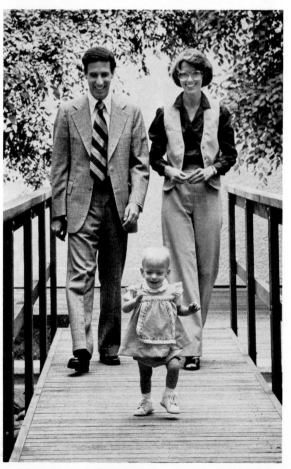

Figure 11. Trailing their exuberant daughter, Sara, Charles and Carolyn return to the hospital for a visit to the nursery. One of the best rewards for professionals in neonatology is seeing a former patient healthy and part of a happy, loving family. Photo by Buster Dean, Houston Chronicle.

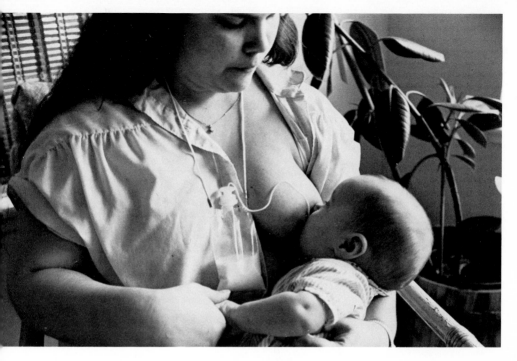

Figure 12. Darleena and her full-term son, Dennis, demonstrate the use of the Lact-Aid Nursing Supplementer. The Lact-Aid encourages increased production of breast milk by providing supplemental formula while also encouraging the baby to continue sucking.
Photo by Craig Stotts.

Figure 13. Steve beams proudly at one of his twin sons, Duncan, who survived a number of complications related to his prematurity, including implantation of a shunt (visible just behind the ear) because of hydrocephalus. Parents often live with nagging fears that prematurity will cause other problems in the future.
Photo by Jeanette Geron.

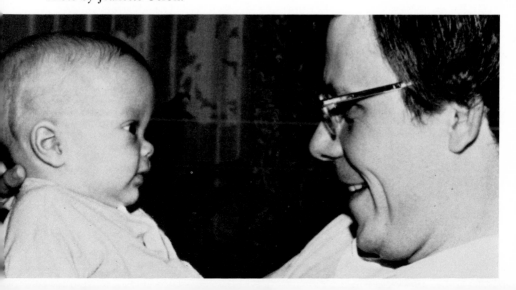

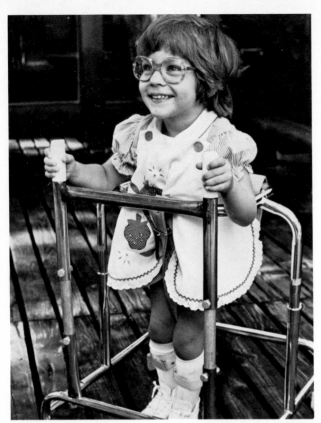

Figure 14. Four year old Angela, a premie who was later diagnosed as having cerebral palsy, is described by her mother as a "self-secure and enthusiastic child who feels few limitations."
Photo by Craig Stotts.

Figure 15.
Photo by Craig Stotts.

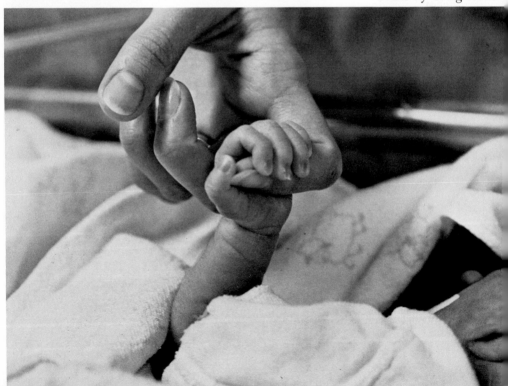

People often ask, "How can anyone have several weeks or months to get things ready and yet not be prepared for the baby to come home?" One reason is that some parents find it difficult to believe that a baby who seems to have been in the hospital "forever" is truly coming home. Others are exhausted from constant trips to the hospital, combined with mental fatigue caused by worry.

In addition, all parents prepare for their babies' homecomings in different ways. Some mothers begin to make baby clothes and to collect baby items from the moment they discover they are pregnant. Fathers may buy toys in anticipation. Other parents wait.

Babies always affect a family's life, but premature infants often seem to their parents to be enormous responsibilities.

COMING HOME, AT LAST

Quite a few parents remember the date their children came home more readily than their birthdays. They recall which nurses were on duty, remember the delays caused by the inevitable hospital red tape and picture again the assembling of baby's leftover medicines, supplies and the complimentary packages of diapers and samples that "new" babies take home. Some reflect apprehensively on times when the baby was "almost" released.

> One day when I arrived at the nursery, the nurses and resident doctor told me that they felt sure that Ryan would be released that day. I couldn't believe it. I waited several hours for Ryan's doctor to make his rounds. When he told me he didn't feel my baby was ready to go home, I was crushed. As it turned out, it was another month until Ryan was released. Thank God, we didn't rush it.

When homecoming day finally does arrive, parents must endure one last hospital policy: "Every infant discharged will be carried to the door by a nurse."

Parents leave with mixed emotions, happy that their infants received the best of care, but jealous that others have had more opportunity to become closely attached to their babies. They may also fear leaving the security they feel when surrounded by the medical staff.

One thing is certain: Homecoming is just as dramatic and emotional a day for parents whose child has been hospitalized for a few extra days as for parents whose child has been hospitalized several weeks or months. In this society, it is not common for newborns to be sick or to remain in the hospital long after birth. Any deviation from the norm is upsetting.

It is not unusual for the homecoming day to come as a surprise to parents. After several "almost" homecomings, Ryan's mother was shocked one day to learn her son was to be released that day:

> Ryan's hospital stay had lasted three long months. During the first week, I had wondered how I could endure being separated from him for even that one week. All but our family and closest friends had stopped asking when he was coming home.
>
> Ryan's problem was not a matter of weight gain. For the last month, he required 1 percent extra oxygen. Without it, he would turn blue and his respiration rate would go up. The doctor talked of the possibility of our bringing him home on oxygen, but as desperately as I wanted him home, I was fearful of that kind of responsibility.
>
> One Monday at 8 a.m., I arrived for Ryan's feeding. The nurses were all smiles. One asked, "Aren't you excited that Ryan is being released this morning?" I was shocked! I learned that the doctor had tried to call me but I was en route to the hospital.
>
> As I waited for my husband to bring Ryan's coming-home outfit, I was excited, but until we got our son in our own car, I was also apprehensive that something else would go wrong.
>
> When we got home, I felt just as I had expected to feel three months earlier—the proud mother arriving home

with her new baby. I wanted to show him off to the whole world. I wanted to shout with joy.

Others have similar stories of the surprise and exhilaration of baby's homecoming.

> I knew that it was almost time for Mindy to come home when she no longer had her milk drip, her monitor, her apnea medicine, her Isolette or gavage feedings; she was now drinking from a bottle in an open crib. For all but the way her clothes fit and her shaved head, she looked like any other baby.
>
> I quit work on Friday, with Mindy weighing 3 pounds and 11 ounces. I thought I had plenty of time to get things ready. On Monday, I was out in the garage painting her dresser when the phone rang. It was her doctor. He said, "Mrs. Wade, how would you like to take your little girl home?" I couldn't believe it. I know I must have stuttered for a full minute or so before answering, "Ah, ah, ah YES!!! When?" The doctor said, "How about today?"
>
> I couldn't wait until Milton could get home. I paced the floor . . . . Wouldn't you know it? He was late because he was out buying me a rocking chair. He came home with a big grin on his face; he was so proud of the rocker. I grabbed him at the door and said, "Yes, it's nice. Let's go get Mindy!"
>
> At the hospital, Milton went to sign her out. Later, he said he hadn't minded at all . . . those were her freedom papers.

As Mindy's mom mentioned, there are clues for watchful parents that a baby is improving and may soon be ready to go home. The most obvious sign is the removal of the medical equipment used for the baby. Other clues include the infant's ability to suck well, gain weight, maintain a stable body temperature and breathe room air; the medical staff's offer to teach parents how to perform special procedures or to allow a mother to breast-feed; the decision to circumcise a baby boy.

Doctors today do not discharge a baby solely on the basis of weight. In the past, 5 pounds seemed to be a magic number, but some babies have gone home weighing only 3 or 4 pounds.

BABY'S HOME! NOW WHAT?

> Inside our house, we walked straight to his nursery. The ritual of placing a new baby in a crib overwhelmed us. In the crib, he seemed so small. It had been too long a struggle to come to think of a 5-pound baby as fat and big.
>
> I had no regrets that my husband had to go back to work. For a while, I wanted my baby to myself. I finally had some time alone with my son and could listen to the music of easy breathing.

Charlie's parents thought that they had left the hospital behind the day their son came home; then came a telephone call:

> Finally we all got into bed . . . . At midnight, the phone rang . . . it was the nursery. They wanted to know, "What does he weigh? What are his respirations? How much did he drink?" All the same things we had called to ask every night at midnight!

The joy of having a baby come home gives way to harsh realities—to isolation, fatigue and occasionally fear.

Isolation

Many doctors advise parents that their babies will require a period of adjustment at home before they should be exposed to the outside world. Parents must remember that their baby has moved from a virtually sterile hospital environment to the "real" world of germs and other potential hazards. Animals, young children, insecticides, pollution and chemicals can be harmful for premies.

Precautions and isolation may be necessary for a period of several weeks. In special circumstances, an isolation period may be extended.

> Because of Ryan's respiratory problems, instead of being able to show off our new son to the world, we came home to nine months of isolation.
>
> Our 2½-year-old demanded that I become very inven-

tive to keep him amused at home. For fear of the contagious illnesses he might bring home, we took him out of
preschool and he seldom saw a friend his own age. The
highlight of his week was going grocery shopping with
me. When we came home, we would both scrub down
before touching baby.

My husband and I longed to go out for an evening
alone but felt we couldn't. I didn't know anyone I felt I
could leave my baby with. He was too unpredictable, and
I was still leery that something could go wrong.

For other parents, the isolation period is not so long, but
precautions are taken when the baby goes out. At times, there
are unexpected consequences for parents.

Monica stayed in the apartment in confinement for exactly four weeks after she came home . . . then I started
carrying her everywhere, but with a few basic rules. No
one was to hold her. No children were to get near her
face. And she and her things were to be as clean as possible. As a result I constantly wiped off the toys Monica
would throw to the ground before returning them to her.

One evening, as she sat in her jump seat next to my
chair at a choir rehearsal, she threw one of her toys for
what must have been the tenth time when one of the
choir members yelled, "Hey look, gang, she's going to do
it again."

I looked up to see the whole choir waiting for me to
wipe off her squeeze toy with a Baby Wipe one more
time. They were teasing, but I turned red and felt very
frustrated.

Monica's godmother, also in the choir, called me the
next day and told me to stick in there, to do whatever I
had to do. She said that none of the other choir members
had had my experiences and that I hadn't had theirs.

She added that it really did seem hysterical to watch
a mother wash off a toy so many times when other mothers have raised a bunch of healthy kids who've probably
eaten their own mud pies and borrowed each other's
pacifiers. But she also said I should never be intimidated
by anyone when trying to do what's right for my child.

A mother who was surprised by unexpected twins had some sound advice for isolated parents or those who have just come home with a new baby:

> You need to take care of yourselves, too. So go to dinner, just the two of you, or go to a show. Take a walk. Strike a comfortable balance between your roles as a parent, a spouse and an individual.

Parents who find nurses or other couples who have cared for a premie and who are willing to baby-sit are among those who feel the most comfortable about going out.

The "Baby Blues"

The delay in taking home a premature infant often means that a mother will experience a similar delay in feeling postpartum depression.

> After Zachary came home, I thought I would have a terminal case of the happies. Instead, the loneliness of isolation and the constant demands of this not-so-new-anymore baby started to affect my moods. I was sad; I was happy. I was tired. I was lonely. I was a mother, but it seemed nobody knew it. I was afraid my fears for Zachary's health would never end.
>   It finally dawned on me I was feeling like most new mothers. Deciding I was behaving normally did much to help me get over the "blues."

Another mother felt a good deal of resentment and frustration after her son came home, sure signs of the "baby blues":

> I did not accept all of this like a true soldier . . . . After the [four] surgeries and Jimmy's problems seemed to be over, I still was not coping . . . . I resented my husband who could walk into the adult world while I felt pinned [at home] with two babies. I felt useless since I [had

previously had] a career as an R.N. and I was not happy
with [diaper-changing] and sick babies. We did not have
family near us . . . so I was feeling sorry for myself a lot.

For others, the severity of the depression is so extreme that
professional care is required. One mother, who was hospitalized
twice for depression, is firm in her conviction that a diagnosis of
the degree of depression is important:

Unlike a cold or flu, it doesn't physically "put you to bed"
the worse it gets. I am thankful my family saw that my
"baby blues" were not a passing feeling and aided me in
seeking the professional help I needed so badly.

Mothers recovering from a difficult delivery and those pumping breast milk are particularly vulnerable to criticism and other
stresses.

Rules

Often, premies go home with rules to meet the medical needs
of their sensitive systems. Such rules are often taxing to follow
and difficult to enforce.

The doctors explained that Mindy needed to wear a hat
to keep her from sunburning; to take multivitamins, iron,
vitamin D and vitamin E; to be kept warm; to be awakened every three hours to eat; to be kept away from kids
or people who were sick; not to be taken out for a while,
etc.

However, some of my relatives did not think the rules
applied to them. One flatly told me, "If my kids can't
come over, then I'm not going to come until they can."
I was very hurt. I wanted to show Mindy off, but I was not
going to beg relatives and friends to come see her.

People can be so cruel or just thoughtless. If they
would stop and think, "What would I do if I were in the
same situation? Would I want someone doing that to
me?"

In looking back at her daugher's early days at home, Mindy's mother had this advice for other parents:

> Do what your physician and common sense tell you. *Be
> a bully. Your baby worked and fought hard to stay here.*
> Let him or her have a chance. You can always make new
> friends if they insist on being mad. Most usually cool
> down and understand the situation better after they are
> given time.

Some parents enforce rules strictly. Restrictions may be relaxed as time passes, but enforcing decisions about visiting, smoking and a host of other things can strain relationships with others.

> We were especially glad we were strict about the "no
> visitors" rule. A neighbor stopped her car in front of the
> house and asked if she might come close to see the baby.
> I hesitated before saying, "No." She then said she had to
> get home anyway, as her young son was ill. We were
> bewildered and angry.

> Even today I do not allow smoking in our home. Ryan's
> lungs were so scarred that I feel he doesn't need anything
> further to aggravate the situation. That winter he came
> home, Grandma could only smoke outside . . . bundled
> up to keep warm!

Health Fears

Parents of premature infants in a sense continue the hospital experience and environment when their baby comes home. Many worry about keeping the house as germ-free as possible and at just the right temperature. Concerns about the baby's health continue.

Many fear crib death or SIDS (sudden infant death syndrome) will take their baby from them.

> I knew enough about SIDS to be terrified of it. Statistics
> show that premature babies, especially males, are the

most susceptible in the first few months of life.

I had witnessed enough apnea spells to have come to associate SIDS with apnea . . . . At that time, it seemed that they both meant the same thing—that the baby could suddenly and inexplicably stop breathing.

After Zachary came home, SIDS was the threat I feared most. Everything else I could control to some degree.

Occasionally, events occur that cause a parent to believe that fears about their baby's health and survival are well-founded.

Mindy had apnea quite often in the hospital. I thought she had outgrown it by the time she came home. The second day she was at home, she was asleep on my lap and I was listening to her breathing. I know that a baby's breathing is erratic, but this time it was different.

I waited what seemed like two minutes for her to breathe, but she didn't. I wanted to scream for Milton but I couldn't. All I could do was grab her and shake her. It woke her up and scared her, and she started breathing again.

What this mother may have observed is periodic breathing, which is apnea without cyanosis. Episodes of periodic breathing are common in the respiration of premature infants.

Another mother who faced a similar situation had to give her daughter artificial respiration.

One Sunday morning, two weeks after our daughter came home, I walked into her room to check on her and discovered that she had stopped breathing and was beginning to turn blue. I was home alone and had no idea what was wrong. After I administered artificial respiration, I called my husband to come take us to the hospital. Thank goodness, I had taken the Red Cross Child Care Class!

Our baby was admitted to the hospital again, this time for viral pneumonia. Ten days later, she came home to a nervous mother. I was sure she would die from crib death or some other horrible thing. I questioned my ability to care for her since I had already "failed" once.

Fatigue

Adjusting to the needs of a premature baby can be tiring. As Trey's mother so aptly put it, "One mother cannot equal three shifts of nurses." Caring for a premie can exhaust both parents. For some of these infants, "schedule" is a nonexistent word.

> His eating and sleeping schedule was a mess! That's the best way to describe it. It seemed like I was always feeding him, and he slept very little. It took him a full year to develop decent sleeping habits.

Determination, a bit of sympathy and help from others, and a sense of humor are indispensable to tired parents. Zachary's mother smiled as she said:

> Many mothers of premies will recognize some of the syndromes that mysteriously appear soon after the baby comes home: "It's past noon and I'm still not dressed yet." "I can hardly wait for my night out at the supermarket." "Oh, Lord, did he—sneeze, cough, sputter, shiver, twitch, cry, whimper, wet or change color?!" "Doctor, this is Mrs.——calling again. I hate to bother you, but. . . ." "He gained a pound? Call everybody!" "That dog, cat, bird, fish, kid . . . is germy; he stays out." *"Husband:* What did you do today, honey? *Wife:* Feed the baby!"

PREMIES AT HOME

While parents must adjust to caring for their baby, the premie also faces adjustments. The infant's still immature nervous system may cause difficult behavior that is puzzling to parents. Frequent feedings are expected, but other problems of adjustment may come as a surprise.

Ryan's mother felt that her son's behavior was also affected by his past negative experiences:

> Ryan came home an uptight, untrusting, tense little boy —with good reason. For three months, whenever someone touched him, it almost always involved pain.

Caring for such an infant is taxing, even for experienced mothers and fathers.

> The frequent feedings, colic and diarrhea were detriments to establishing good sleeping habits. Also, when Karen learned to stand up she couldn't figure out how to sit down. At night, I would often make four or five trips to her room.
>
> Overall, she was *not* a happy baby. With each milestone of infancy (crawling, sitting, standing and walking), Karen became happier, however. At about eighteen months of age, she finally began acting "human," sleeping through the night and enjoying things and people around her.

Not all premies are temperamental babies. There are, however, other problems related to their prematurity. Some become ill within a few weeks or months after leaving the hospital, or other medical problems appear. Karen, for example, returned to the hospital with viral pneumonia after two weeks at home. Then came other complications:

> Karen's X rays were looking better, but the doctor warned us that another bout with a respiratory problem would be serious. Therefore, we extended our isolation time longer than we had planned. She and her brother Bobby were kept in separate rooms when he was home, and we wore masks if we had colds.
>
> To complicate matters, Karen began having severe colic. This took me completely by surprise since she was 2½ months old. I had always associated colic with newborns. The doctor informed me that colic doesn't show

up in premature babies until two to four weeks after the due date. So we suffered through colic for nearly four months at which time she began having diarrhea.

By this time, I was beginning to feel like an old hand at children's illnesses, but I had never before dealt with nonspecific diarrhea.

From May until October, Karen was on and off diarrhea diets, at which time I had had it. She was hospitalized again to be tested for malabsorption. After three days of tests, the results were negative. So we were back to square one: nonspecific diarrhea.

Premies' systems are often still immature when they come home. Not understanding the effects of this immaturity can cause confusion and frustration for parents trying their best to give proper care and love to their baby.

Under Special Circumstances

Special precautions or procedures may be necessary if a baby comes home with a handicap or a long-term medical difficulty. These problems can range from allergies to respiratory difficulties to mental or physical disabilities. Although these special circumstances will be covered more thoroughly in chapter nine, it is important to note that the required therapy or treatment usually has an unsettling effect on a household. A mother whose son came home with oxygen for emergencies and a schedule of inhalation therapy three times a day gave an insight into the changes that her baby brought to his new home:

I kept a Lysol house for months and sterilized everything possible. After shopping I even considered my clothing contaminated, so I would change before touching the baby.

We all had the healthiest, cold-free year I could remember. But I lived in fear of Ryan or any of us getting sick. Until his lungs got larger and stronger, I was so afraid of what a simple cold could mean for him.

It is important that a child be exposed to common colds

to build up some resistance; however, with a premie who has had severe respiratory problems, you want the exposure to come gradually. A child is going to get a cold sooner or later. I hoped for later.

The specialized care some premies receive while hospitalized can be disconcerting to parents when they bring their baby home. They may take even greater precautions to assure that the child will survive and do well under their care. For example, some parents ask that their child have a heart monitor at home, which usually is relinquished once they begin to feel secure. Because of Victor's many episodes of apnea and bradycardia, his mother said:

> So we took home our beautiful little baby and one heart-apnea monitor. And we became slaves to a machine.
>
> The monitor consisted of a belt with sensors that fit around Victor's chest. The belt was attached to the box via long wires . . . . Two lights flashed on the monitor. One light blinked in response to Victor's breathing; the other recorded his heart rate.
>
> An alarm would sound if Victor either stopped breathing for a certain number of seconds or if his heart rate fell below a certain number of beats per minute.
>
> Numerous times during the day and night, I would glance at the lights and then at Victor just to be sure. But we never heard an alarm.
>
> After two or three weeks I managed to say, "This is craziness. God forgive me." I packed the monitor in its box and turned it in at the end of the month.

Keeping Records

An isolated mother may imagine her baby has had a problem like diarrhea forever, when in reality it has been two days. Notes can keep track of specific behavior that may indicate illness or developmental difficulties. Parents who find note-taking useful should continue doing so until they feel comfortable not keeping records. Records can include such information as:

1. Ounces of formula consumed at each feeding, or feeding schedule if breast-feeding.
2. Any worrisome behavior, such as listlessness or a sudden or extreme change in the baby's sleeping or eating patterns.
3. Signs of possible illness, such as breathing difficulties, fever, vomiting, any unusual discharge or bowel movements, constipation or extreme diarrhea.
4. Developmental activity (rolling over, new teeth, smiling, etc.).

DAY-TO-DAY LIFE

In addition to the serious problems that parents of premies encounter, they also discover some challenging and amusing aspects, like finding tiny clothes and adapting baby products.

Buying Clothes

Not many parents have a toddler who can go through two winters with the same coat because the child remains small. And how many parents can say that their twelve-month-old can still wear newborn-size disposable diapers? One woman said, "When any mother started the pity routine about my kids' small sizes, I'd tell her that I was getting more for my money than she was. Newborn-size diapers are less expensive than larger diapers, and my kids wore newborns for a year!" Some gowns, T-shirts and layette sets can be comfortably worn by a premie for a year or more, making the cost of the baby's clothing quite reasonable.

In the past few years, stores across the country have begun to stock ready-to-wear premie-size clothes, which appeared on the market in response to appeals to manufacturers and individuals by parents of premies and parent support groups. (A list of such manufacturers and individuals is included in Resources, page 000.)

As the child grows, parents may find that the usual designations of size by age are confusing. Often it is best to shop with the baby, but it is also helpful for shoppers to know how size designations by age relate to weight and height. The following chart gives weight and height figures for standard sizes:

size	pounds	inches
3 mos.	13	24
6 mos.	18	26½
12 mos.	22	29
18 mos.	26	31½
24 mos.	29	34
36 mos.	32	36½
1 toddler	25	31
2 toddler*	29	34
3 toddler*	34	37
4 toddler*	38	40

*Body measurements for toddler sizes 2, 3 and 4 are the same for children's sizes 2, 3 and 4. Toddler sizes are cut fuller to fit children still in diapers and those who still have their "baby fat."

Adapting Baby Products

When infants first come home, their small size often forces parents to construct many make-do alternatives to the usual baby products. Car seats to take the baby home in begin the cycle.

> When I put Zachary in the car seat, he vanished for a moment. Then, there he was, this rag doll, lost in a sea of black vinyl. Boy, was I irritated. Who did they design these baby products for anyway, Baby Huey?
>
> I finally lined the seat with two zipped comforters. They were soft, sort of like a nest. They added enough bulk so that the seat belt fit properly. I held his head in place with rolled baby blankets. He looked like a wiener in a hot-dog bun, but he was safe.

Susan's parents discovered a combination infant carrier and car seat, the Dyn-O-Mite by Questor, that was easy to adapt for their daughter. Others have recommended the Strolee Wee Care car seat, the GM Love Seat, the Peterson Safety Shell and the Bobby Mac 3-in-1 car seat (without a deceleration shield). For any of these, a supply of receiving blankets or towels is needed to provide additional padding.

Because of the infant's small size, many parents decide that cradles or bassinets are more appropriate beds than full-size cribs. The rocking of a cradle sometimes calms a fussy infant, and most small babies seem to prefer a cozy place to sleep and play. One mother found that the carriage she had intended to use outside made a useful, and portable, short-term bed for her baby. Small babies can also sleep comfortably in laundry baskets, plastic infant bathtubs or drawers from a chest outfitted with a foam mattress.

Bumper pads for cribs are absolute necessities. A small baby's head can slip between the side rails for many months. In some instances, the entire baby can fall through the rails!

Several parents mentioned that at times when their babies were particularly irritable, one effective way of getting their infants to fall asleep was to use what one parent described as a "living mattress." The technique involves putting the child on a mother's or father's chest or stomach and gently patting the baby's back or bottom until both parent and child fall asleep. Somehow none of the parents ever rolled over to send their babies tumbling.

Other parents have found that bringing the child to their bed is calming. For safety, some parents put the baby in a small basket or baby bathtub that is placed at the head of the bed between the parents.

During the day, strap-on infant carriers often prove handy for busy mothers. The close contact and constant movement helps comfort colicky or fussy babies. One manufacturer, Snugli, has developed the Premie Snugli® available through some retail outlets or from Resources in Human Nurturing International. (See Resources, page 000, for the address.) This organization also sells lambskins, which have been popular infant care products in New Zealand and Australia for years. The soft wool is said to provide tactile stimulation as well as to help babies sleep better and longer. Both infant carriers and lambskins are used in some NICUs.

Parents who decide to purchase high chairs, walkers, swings and other items are confronted by the size problem.

Have you ever tried to find a walker for a 2-foot-tall baby? Many that I looked at were so high off the floor that not even her toes would have touched the ground!

Finally, one sympathetic saleswoman understood my problem. She showed me the kind she had purchased as a gift for her premature niece. It was called the Super-coupe, made by Century Products. It can be adjusted to as little as 6 inches off the floor.

Putting a small baby in a high chair is often impossible for many months, although the baby may be eating solid foods and teething on crackers or toast. Many parents have found that an infant carrier placed in an upright position is a good substitute for a high chair. If unable to sit unsupported, the baby's head may need to be propped with rolled towels or receiving blankets.

For feeding, it is useful to have on hand a supply of 4-ounce bottles and premie nipples since at first the baby will not be able to drink an entire 8-ounce bottle. Because a breast-fed premie may need supplemental feedings, small-size bottles are also convenient for nursing mothers. Premixed formula may be purchased in small cans or ready-to-use bottles. Formula in larger cans may be wasted since, for several weeks at least, the baby will not drink all of the formula within the time span indicated on the label. Premie nipples and Nuk nipples, which some mothers feel are easier for their babies to suck, may be purchased in some local and hospital pharmacies or ordered through a pharmacist. Regular nipples can be crosscut to allow milk to flow more freely, but care should be taken so that the nipple opening is not too big.

Another product that parents have reported to be useful is a bouncing infant chair. To a small baby, the chair is like a miniature hammock, and most babies, fussy or not, love it!

When sufficiently developed for a wind-up baby swing, a premie may still be too small and light. Many parents find it necessary to weight and pad the swing seat so it does not swing too fast. A clean brick, book or other small, heavy object wrapped in a towel and topped by padding makes a comfortable seat. The baby can be secured by loosely tying a folded receiving blanket under the arms and around the seat back.

Some wind-up swings have a bassinet attachment. The rhythmic movement of the bassinet may soothe a tense baby and make the infant sleepy. A swinging bassinet, like the seat of a wind-up swing, must be weighted to prevent too rapid swinging. Rolled blankets can be tucked around a small baby to keep the infant in place.

An excellent source of information on baby products is *The Complete Baby Book* by the editors of *Consumers Guide* (New York: Simon and Schuster, 1979).

Caring for Baby

There are challenges in living with any new baby. But more are encountered by parents who bring home babies that were born prematurely.

Bath time can be quite an experience. One mother, who was the oldest of six children and had bathed infants many times, found that the bathtub was so large in comparison to her child that it was a "pool" where she could teach her little one how to float. Another mother, on the other hand, said:

> Even though it was summer, Zachary would become chilled in his bath. It was like a marathon race to get him undressed, into the warm water and out again.
>
> Meanwhile, he screamed as I'd never heard him scream in the hospital. Until he was dried and wrapped warmly in a towel, his skin would remain a mottled red and white for a while.
>
> Eventually, he came to love his bath given in a large plastic salad bowl.

Mothers whose infants dislike bath time may wish to try the following suggestions that other mothers of premies have found helpful:

1. Distract the baby with music or a toy.
2. Bathe the baby in front of a mirror. The reflection may be fascinating enough that the baby forgets the bath.

3. Leave the baby partially dressed; a slip-on infant shirt works well.
4. Use an inflatable bathtub or a sponge insert for an infant bathtub.
5. Change the lighting level to see if the baby prefers bright or subtle light.
6. Alter the temperature of the bathwater or the room, but avoid chilling a small baby.
7. Ask another person for help. A father or grandparent may work wonders at bath time.

One universal difficulty for parents of premies seems to be the infants' adjustment to a world of "night" and "day." In the hospital nursery, the child has known only twenty-four hours of light and may not associate sleeping with nighttime. Parents who have dealt with the day/night reversal offered the following suggestions:

1. Keep baby on a strict three- or four-hour feeding schedule during the day; allow the infant to sleep at night.
2. To avoid fatigue, sleep when the baby sleeps.
3. If the baby becomes tired after a bath, bathe at night. If a bath makes the baby alert, bathe during the day.
4. Try taking the baby for a walk or a ride in the car. The constant motion of a wind-up swing may lull the baby to sleep. A rocking chair may be helpful.
5. Experiment with nursery lighting—use a night-light or install a dimmer control in baby's room. Try various temperature settings and background noises—a radio, music box or ticking clock. Some sounds are especially soothing to a baby; others are disturbing. Find which ones your baby prefers.

Many mothers have found that a slightly noisy house helps their premies adjust to the new environment. The vacuum cleaner seems to be one machine that matches the dull roar of the incubator. Instead of being startled, many premies fall asleep to the sound. Other mothers have had similar success running cold-mist humidifiers. For some, nothing seems to help.

> Our daughter started sleeping through the night with regularity at [about] 2½. One premie I am familiar with [had], at the age of three years, slept through the entire night only nine times. Our daughter is 3½, . . . and she still often wakes at least once during the night.

There are other, somewhat ordinary aspects of caring for a new baby that are slightly modified for the premie. For example, inoculations against childhood diseases are usually delayed a few months past recommended dates. A baby boy may not have been circumcised, as the procedure may have been considered too stressful. Like babies born at term, premies have their own individual temperaments and unique requirements.

A Special Note

Surveys have shown that child abuse is more frequent among children who were born prematurely. There are certain aspects of dealing with a premie that, if understood, may help parents cope with the frustration these babies can cause.

1. A premature infant's cry is physiologically different from that of a full-term baby. The crying of a premie may be more frequent and high-pitched.
2. A premie can be "disorganized," overly active or irritable. Fussiness is often a result of unintentional overstimulation. A parent who rocks, pats and sings to a premie—all at the same time—may be greeted with crying from an upset child who the parent believes is being comforted.
3. Separation from a hospitalized infant in the first weeks or months of life may affect in a negative way the relationship between the parent and the child. It may take parents time to understand their own feelings about the experience.

4. A child who has long-range problems or who has undergone numerous medical procedures may not smile as often as other babies or seem as happy as other infants. An unresponsive child can cause parents to become unresponsive.

It is normal to feel periodically frustrated or angry with any child, either because of the child's actions, clashes of personality or outside events. If a parent's response is potentially harmful to the child, the parent should seek help immediately from relatives, friends, a local crisis hotline or Parents Anonymous. (See Resources, page 000.)

Parenting classes and discussion groups are often valuable in helping parents understand their child's behavior and their own reactions to certain behavior.

KEEPING IN TOUCH WITH PROFESSIONALS

It is important to contact the baby's pediatrician or the family doctor when questions about the baby's health arise, but it may be particularly helpful in easing parents' worries if they can contact a social worker, special nurse, intern or doctor from the nursery when they need advice or have questions.

Also, doctors and nurses usually enjoy receiving periodic progress reports on the infants they have brought through their perilous early days. It gives them a boost to see that the children are loved and doing well. Some hospitals encourage parents to send in photographs after the baby comes home for a nursery bulletin board or sponsor reunions for graduates of special care units and their parents.

This relationship between parents and professionals is beneficial to both sides. The staff feel pride and a sense of accomplishment; the parents feel secure knowing that the doctors and nurses will give honest, objective advice.

FIRST OUTINGS

Parents know their baby is truly home when they begin to take their child on outings. For some parents, it is at this time that many worries are alleviated. A premie's first trip out is usually to a doctor's office and is not an outing in the true sense. Nonetheless, it is a memorable experience.

Two weeks after Mindy's release, we made our first visit to the pediatrician and to the pediatric ophthalmologist. I was excited about being able to show her off, but at the same time frightened by the idea of getting my baby out in the germy world.

Taking her to the pediatrician's office was not too bad. We went straight to the examining room to wait for the doctor in private. I realized the pediatrician must have told everyone about Mindy when all the nurses came in to see her. One nurse made a comment I have never forgotten, "How can something so small be so perfect?"

I was not at all looking forward to going to the pediatric ophthalmologist's office. It was on the twenty-second floor, and we would have to park in the fumey, gassy, polluted covered garage.

The elevator ride up was not too bad . . . there were only two other people. They said, "Oh, what a little baby! How old is she? How much does she weigh?" "Four pounds and 7 ounces and 3½ months old." I knew I would hear this a lot, but I was thankful my floor had come up.

After the examination, I carried Mindy into the hall and we got on the elevator again. As it went down, more and more people got on. It was so crowded!

I didn't like exposing my daughter to so many people —and germs—at one time. Although I was as proud as any mother and wanted to show her off, when someone asked to see her, I said, "She's asleep" and held her close to me. I was tired and didn't want to have to answer any more questions.

If a family has endured a lengthy isolation period, going out for dinner or to a park are delightful moments.

I am not an overprotective mother, but Charlie's respiratory problems kept us temporary prisoners of our house. Finally at fourteen months, we took Charlie out to eat. (Of course, we went during the week when more people stay home.) He practically broke his neck looking at all the people and the lights.

I said, "Hey Charlie, there's a whole new world that I want to show you. Hang in there, honey, and we'll get to it as soon as you are able."

If grandparents live out of town or in another state, that first trip to grandma's house can be quite an experience. Parents become accustomed to common remarks and questions. One mother listed what parents should expect to hear:

They all remarked: "How cute he is!" "Isn't it a miracle he is alive?" "When will he catch up physically?" "Will he be all right?" "Is he sickly?" and "Isn't it a miracle he is alive!"

The repetition can become boring, but it also allows parents the opportunity to talk about their experiences and their feelings.

Ryan's mother told a tale of travel with an unusual twist:

When Ryan was a year old, we took him back to California to meet his relatives. Everyone was hesitant to touch or hold him or to ask or say much about him.

My warnings for "anyone with so much as a sniffle" to stay away had had its impact. I expected my family to be ready to receive him with open arms, to cuddle and caress him. Not so. Everyone was apprehensive and a little bit afraid. The idea of his inhalation therapy was a scary thought to my relatives and our friends.

I was particularly disappointed that no one was willing to watch Ryan even for an evening so my husband and I could go out alone.

Then a close friend of mine, a nurse, came to visit. She cuddled, caressed and jostled with him. She reassured me of how normal and healthy he was. I don't know if she'll ever realize how important that message was to me at that time. I was finally able to show off my son after we had received a very standoffish reception.

A year later my family had warmed up considerably to our rough, tough two-year-old son.

PREMIE STORIES

It seems that all parents of premies hear an abundance of premie stories after their child's birth. Just as the woman who learns she is pregnant suddenly begins to notice every other pregnant woman, parents of a premie either notice exceptionally small babies, are recognized as having a premie by other parents or are told about other premies by well-meaning acquaintances.

Once parents and baby are going out together, chance encounters with other parents of premature infants are likely. These encounters can be touching or unnerving.

While shopping one evening, a stranger practically ran to me as I put my daughter into the shopping basket. This woman asked, "Can I please see your baby?" as she tried to hug my daughter. I was hesitant, but for some reason I sensed a desperate need in her.

She asked how old my child was and I answered, "Five months." I don't know why the good Lord brought us together at that moment, but it happened that the woman had lost a premature son in the same hospital where I delivered, within a week of my having had twins and losing our son.

I had taken a job again in a neighborhood bank to help with the financial obligations resulting from Trey's birth and for personal reasons.

On one day, business was slow, which allowed time for friendly conversations with the customers. A soft, gray-haired woman placing money back in her wallet flipped through to a picture of an adorable baby boy about Trey's age. Upon seeing it, I commented on how cute and how proud she must be of that grandbaby.

Then she proceeded to tell me the story of this darling child. He had been two months early as Trey had been, hospitalized for several months as Trey had been, recovered and gone home and began to do well as Trey had. With each of these points, we talked of the similarities.

Her next remark was that he had died unexpectedly at eighteen months of age. I was sad and sick for her at her loss, but it also aroused in me feelings I thought to be dead and buried.

I wanted to drop everything I was doing, get Trey and go to every possible source for reassurance that this last point would not also become a similarity. This panicky, desperate feeling remained for a while; earlier fears of Trey's first days and those first months at home surfaced again.

However, as before, time hammered things back in order.

THE END, THE BEGINNING OR STUCK IN THE MIDDLE?

Once the baby has been released from the hospital and can finally go out among people, parents feel the excitement and pride of having a "new" baby. After weeks or months of hospitalization, and sometimes isolation, parents and their premies are at a point that full-term infants and their parents usually reach within a week or so after birth.

Despite the joy, parents may also be frustrated by other people's comments. Mothers of healthy babies ask how it is that this child, the size of her three-month-old, is able to sit up in the basket and play with the groceries! Indignant grandmothers ask, "Why is this newborn outside?" Parents should reconcile themselves to the facts: A sixteen-month-old baby born prematurely may have the aptitude of an eighteen-month-old, the physical abilities of a thirteen-month-old and the size of somebody's four-month-old. It is a part of the experience of prematurity.

> Someday you finally quit having to explain. When someone says, "She's so small," you reply, "Yes, she is," and you don't feel the need to continue.
> The biggest breakthrough for me came when someone invariably asked, "Do you have any others?" and I didn't

have to reply, "No, but we lost her twin."

From then on, I was more secure. Monica was no longer the child who had been in the hospital eighty days, had had two operations and had weighed 2 pounds and 3 ounces at her lowest weight, but Monica who could run and stumble and throw her toys with the best of 'em.

Wait—I'm Not Ready!
(Thoughts of a mother of a premature infant)

The pain moves in waves,
Rhythmically pushing out what too recently
Began to grow in me.
A nameless lump just beginning to show itself,
Now, too early, to enter the world as my own . . .

> *Wait—I'm not ready!*

A tiny dark figure
Gasping for his first breath in a cold world,
Laboring silently at the business of survival,
Too small, too unfinished, too soon.
And now I'm a mother . . .

> *Wait—I'm not ready!*

Alone in my room,
Despite happy laughs from behind the curtain,
Listening to the cries of babes of other mothers,
Wondering if it all has really happened,
And carrying not my child but cards and flowers . . .

> *Wait—I'm not ready!*

In the midst of lights and tubes and wires,
Buzzers, bells, dials and gauges,
I've come to introduce myself to my baby, intruding.
Past the other bodies—babies—living victims encased
*   in plastic;*
> *Mine can't be like those.*
Oh God! This one can't be mine!

Wait—I'm not ready!

Waiting, watching at his side,
He dreams of floating, rocking in wet warmth.
I dream of nursing, nurturing a warm bundle, nuzzling
*   at my breast.*
But it's not meant to be; not yet.
I'm mother to one still a stranger . . .

Wait—I'm not ready!

At last, together in our home
He sleeps in my arms, wrapped in stripes of blue
*   and white.*
He's found his place so late for one so early,
And now I know the gift that came to me.
My chance, my turn to learn to love . . .

I'm ready.

Lauri Lowen

Chapter 8

FEEDING
A PREMIE

The question of how a baby will be fed, whether by bottle or breast, is one that all parents must answer eventually. The feeding of a premature infant is not a simple matter of choice, however. There are factors to be weighed that generally are not considered when an infant is born at term. Some of these considerations are medical; some are personal. On occasion, compromises regarding initial decisions about feeding must be made.

Often when a baby is born prematurely, the medical staff encourages the mother to pump her breasts to provide milk for her baby. Most mothers view pumping as their unique contribution to the care of their babies. Those who had not intended to breastfeed often change their minds when the matter of feeding is discussed with them. Others, however, may resent being placed in the position of feeling that they must do something they never wanted to do.

A MATTER OF CHOICE, SOMETIMES

Some parents prefer to bottle-feed their babies. Some mothers wish to breast-feed but encounter difficulties with the pumping, freezing, storing and transporting necessary to get milk to the hospital. Some mothers may not breast-feed for medical reasons.

> I had no choice about bottle-feeding my son. . . . Charlie had such severe respiratory problems that it was physically impossible for him to take more than 2 ounces every three hours. Sometimes the problems would necessitate gavage feeding, after his turning blue with bottle-feeding, [even] at 6½ pounds.
>
> I do not feel my son was deprived of any bonding because the milk in his drip or bottle was "man-made" and not "mother-made" . . . . He missed the initial antibodies and immunities and that upset me.
>
> I tried to work even harder to make up for the fact that I was not allowed to breast-feed. I held Charlie in a position exactly like nursing. I would raise my shirt and put him on my skin. I would change sides as [though] I [were] changing breasts.
>
> I do not feel I was any less of a mother or woman because my son's sustenance came from a bottle and not my breast.

Experiences regarding decisions on feeding premies occur in endless variations. Occasionally the mother intends to pump and breast-feed, but receives no support from either her husband or her doctors and eventually must decide for herself. Sometimes the mother has had no intent to nurse and is influenced by the doctors.

> The nurse asked me in the labor room whether I was going to breast-feed or bottle-feed. There was never any question for me about this: I definitely was going to bottle-feed. I had always thought that primitive people were the only ones to breast-feed. How vulgar it looked!
>
> The nurse told me she would give me an estrogen shot in the delivery room. After the babies were born, the

pediatrician came into recovery and told me the shot had not been given. He then said he thought it would be best if I could pump my milk and take it to the babies. Naturally, I wanted to do anything to help.

THE CHOICE: BOTTLE-FEEDING

A number of problems may make breast-feeding inadvisable— a mother's ill health, either temporary or chronic, or her need for certain medications that would pass through breast milk to the baby. The health of the infant is another factor. A lactose intolerance, weight loss or the inability to gain weight are some reasons infants are placed on a low-density, high-calorie formula. The higher number of calories per volume of the formula in comparison to breast milk can either assist the infant in gaining ounces more quickly or place less strain on an already taxed gastrointestinal system. As one mother stated:

> This formula should be considered medicine, not food, for a tiny baby whose life depends on how and how much he is fed.

Logistic problems can temporarily or permanently necessitate that a mother bottle-feed. A woman who holds a job, has several other children or lives a great distance from the hospital has special difficulties that may interfere with a milk supply. The added stress of the infant's hospitalization can cause a mother's milk production to decrease drastically.

> I really wanted to breast-feed my baby. The pediatrician encouraged me, and I rented an electric breast pump. Every three hours around the clock I was on the machine. But by the end of five weeks, I was getting less than an ounce a pumping and the baby was taking more.
> This was really frustrating because the only mothering I felt I was doing was the breast-feeding. I was failing at that. Why? I'm not sure but with running to and from the hospital, naps were impossible. I had hardly any appetite and had to force down well-balanced meals. Finally per-

haps emotional fatigue had something to do with it.

I do know that once I realized I wasn't going to be able to continue there was a weight lifted off me. I then put more energy into fixing up the nursery and visiting the hospital rather than worrying whether I was getting enough milk or what I was doing wrong.

There are many cases where the baby can tolerate breast milk and the mother can produce it but the mother decides to bottle-feed. This often occurs due to the difficulties faced by the mother in balancing the extreme stress of the infant's hospitalization and attempts at normalizing her own and her family's life. Even more frequently, a nursing mother may opt to nurse and supplement, due to the numerous difficulties involved in the full-time breast-feeding of a premie.

The mother who makes such a choice for nonmedical reasons should realize there are also difficulties encountered in bottle-feeding a premie. Feedings are frequent, whether nursing or bottle-feeding. Much time may be spent sterilizing bottles, mixing formulas or finding a special type of formula. Bottle-feeding can be tiring, too!

Finding nipples best suited to a premie's need can be difficult. If the baby has a weak sucking reflex, a supply of "premie" nipples is a necessity. They may be obtained upon dismissal from the nursery or purchased at local or hospital pharmacies. Mothers who are bottle-feeding or supplementing may find it helpful to use the brands of nipples that more closely resemble a mother's own.

Another problem with bottle-feeding is that parents have a tendency to become overconcerned about the child's feeding patterns as a result of being able to see the exact amount consumed. In the hospital, where every cc at each feeding is recorded, parents become accustomed to the idea that the infant "should" take a prescribed amount of formula. An infant's appetite varies, just as an adult's does; the "correct" amount varies from feeding to feeding. Some babies may prefer to take smaller amounts of formula more frequently.

THE CHOICE: BREAST-FEEDING

Many neonatologists encourage mothers to pump milk because the immunities and trace elements that are present in colostrum and breast milk compensate in some ways for the natural immunity factors that premies usually lack. These immune factors are especially important to premies, who are susceptible to infections. Another advantage of breast milk to a premie with an immature digestive system is its digestibility.

Michael's mother found that nursing was comforting to her son when he developed severe colic:

> When colic developed, nursing helped us all through the six months of baby discomfort. We would often nurse for two hours at a sitting, alternating breasts every twenty minutes. I would sometimes feel three let-downs in each breast at a feeding. And at the end of two hours, the milk would still stream.
>
> One of my pediatricians was disturbed when I mentioned the nursing times and told me not to nurse more than thirty minutes total at any sitting. He claimed there was never enough milk for any longer period and that if I still had milk it only meant that my baby was not strong enough to suck it out. Not true—for the amount of time my baby sucked, his tummy would show how full he was, and we had a corresponding number of very wet diapers. He also gained weight on nothing but my milk so it was evident that he was getting it. The warmth of my body, of a baby water bottle, and the comfort of nursing did ease the colic discomfort quite a bit. . . .
>
> As soon as the colic subsided, chronic diarrhea began. Or as the doctor diagnosed it, Chronic Nonspecific Infant Intestinal Disorder. It also lasted for many months . . . weight gain continued, but my baby probably ate double the amount necessary to gain half as much.

The decision to provide breast milk can have emotional benefits for the mother.

Breast-feeding is a major factor in helping to span the
gap between a hospitalized baby and a frustrated mother
who wants so desperately to be a part of her baby's life.
It is a tremendous uplift to know that you are making a
contribution to your baby's well-being. A father, too can
take heart in his wife's accomplishments and efforts in
breast-feeding. After all, breast milk is (almost) free. Formula costs money!

Difficulties may arise, however, when a mother attempts to
pump and breast-feed her premature baby. Among the major
problems are the lack of nipple preparation, establishing and
maintaining a proper milk supply with a breast pump, establishing the let-down reflex, an uncooperative baby, a baby with a
weak sucking reflex and the baby's adjustment from bottle-feeding to breast-feeding. These problems may convince even the
most pro–breast-feeding mother to turn to bottle-feeding.

PUMPS AND PUMPING METHODS

Until a mother is able to nurse her baby, breast milk may be
obtained by hand expression or the use of a manual or electric
breast pump.

Here is a list of the methods by which breast milk may be
obtained and the types of pumps currently available, along with
suggestions on how to make the experience a little less difficult
and a little more enjoyable. With any method of pumping, always
start with clean hands, clean breasts (clear, warm water is sufficient to cleanse breasts), clean or sterile pump and sterile container for collecting the milk.

Hand Expression

Massage the breast for a minute or so. Then grasp the breast
with thumb above and fingers below. Compress the areola,
squeezing milk into a container.

Advantages: No cost, very sanitary.

Disadvantages: May be tiring, somewhat difficult to build milk supply.

Manual Pump Expression

RUBBER BULB PUMP. The simplest, most commonly found type of manual pump is the rubber bulb or bicycle horn pump. It consists of a rubber bulb at one end and a hard plastic container at the other end with a small indentation in the plastic container for collecting the milk. When the indentation is filled with milk, it must be emptied before pumping can be resumed. One brand (Evenflo) collects milk directly into a bottle.

To clean the bicycle horn pump, wash it in hot, soapy water, squeezing water in and out of the bulb, too. Rinse thoroughly in the same way under hot running water. Do not boil this type of pump, but you may pour boiling water over or immerse the hard plastic part. If the pump loses its suction, get a new one.

To use this pump, moisten the breast to form better suction. Then attach the pump by squeezing air from the bulb and placing the plastic container over the nipple to form a suction. Repeat to milk the breast.

Advantages: Inexpensive, lightweight, portable and readily available.

Disadvantages: May be difficult to use, somewhat difficult to build milk supply, may be hard on breasts and nipples, sterilization can shorten pump's life span and milk can get into the bulb.

KANESON BREAST MILKING/FEEDING UNIT. This manual pump consists of a long, hard, clear plastic cylinder with a shield at one end. A second cylinder fits inside the first and suction is formed by pulling out the second cylinder like a syringe. The unit holds about 3 ounces and may be converted directly into a feeding unit by attaching a nipple to one end.

Advantages: Simple, efficient, comfortable, lightweight, portable, easy to clean, reasonably priced, good suction.

Disadvantages: Not readily available in some areas, gasket needs to remain dry for proper suction and may wear out easily.

THE LOYD-B PUMP. Another manual pump, the Loyd-B, consists of a pistol-type mechanism, a replaceable glass collection bottle and a replaceable glass shield. The shield is put to the breast in a manner similar to that used with the bicycle horn pump, and the intensity of the suction is regulated by the manual action of the vacuum release trigger.

Advantages: Reasonably priced, efficient, easy to use.

Disadvantages: Glass shield, container or pistol mechanism may break.

Electric Pump Expression

ELECTRIC PUMP. This type of pump consists of an electrically operated suction pump that is attached to a plastic or glass shield and collection container. The electric pump mechanically pulls the breast and releases it in a motion that is similar to that of the sucking of an infant.

Advantages: Very efficient, easier to establish and maintain milk supply, adjustable suction, may be rented, most mothers who use this type of pump prefer it above all others.

Disadvantages: Very expensive to purchase and somewhat expensive to rent, heavy and not very portable, not as readily available as other pumps.

Note: Some insurance companies will pay for the use of an electric pump or the purchase of a Loyd-B pump if prescribed by a doctor.

Tips on Pumping

1. Relax and get plenty of rest.
2. Begin pumping as soon as possible after delivery, preferably within the first twenty-four hours.
3. At first, pump every two to three hours beginning with three minutes on each side and gradually increasing the pumping time to about ten minutes per side. With sore nipples, it may be easier to pump three minutes a side and then repeat for a total of six minutes on each side.

4. After the breasts and nipples have toughened up, pump every two to four hours or as often as needed to supply the quantity of milk required. More frequent pumpings are preferable to longer ones for building milk supply and avoiding sore nipples.
5. Pumping at night is not required unless there is a need to relieve full breasts or to build milk supply.
6. Massage the breasts while using a pump to help empty them completely.
7. Match the pumping schedule to baby's regular feeding schedule.
8. Pump whenever let-down is felt; this is positive reinforcement for the body.

ESTABLISHING THE LET-DOWN REFLEX AND A MILK SUPPLY

In a normal nursing situation, milk is "let down" from storage spaces known as sinuses through the many milk ducts in the breast shortly after the baby begins sucking or when the mother anticipates a regular feeding time. Some mothers describe the let-down of milk as a tingling sensation; others cannot tell when this involuntary action occurs.

When using a pump, it is often difficult to establish a pattern for the let-down reflex. Any tension or stress can inhibit let-down.

Some women find it helpful to stimulate the let-down reflex before applying the pump shield or before putting baby to the breast. Here are some tips on ways to relax and help initiate let-down before pumping or nursing:

1. Place a warm washcloth on the breasts.
2. Gently massage around the breasts and stimulate the nipples.
3. Call the hospital nursery and ask about your baby.
4. Concentrate on a photograph of your baby.
5. Try pumping immediately after visiting your baby.
6. Drink a small glass of liquid to help relax.
7. Take a warm bath or shower.

8. Go outside or for a short walk.
9. Take a nap.
10. Listen to some favorite music or read a good book while pumping.
11. Take two or three deep cleansing breaths.
12. Ask the doctor about a prescription for oxytocin nasal spray to help trigger let-down.

Although it is difficult to relax when your baby is hospitalized, try to stay as calm as possible.

One first time mother describes her difficulty in establishing the let-down reflex:

> I thought I would go crazy trying to experience the elusive let-down required for producing breast milk. Experienced nursing mothers would describe it as a tingling sensation or a pins-and-needles feeling or a heavy, warm fullness of the breasts. Another said it felt like the breast was going to sneeze.
>
> Pumping did not provide that let-down feeling for me. I felt I was clawing the milk out of my breasts. I remember getting so angry at my body for not functioning "normally" that I slapped my breasts with my hands. I do not recommend that. I'd try to rationalize and then imagine what the let-down reflex felt like. I knew that was the key. I considered that let-down must be like an orgasm of the breasts. Trying to think erotic thoughts while pumping didn't help at all.
>
> Then I thought it might help if I used the natural force of gravity to help the milk let-down. So I experimented with pumping while I lay with my head on the floor and my feet on the bed, upside down! Of course, that didn't work.
>
> I pumped sitting in a bath of warm water and after drinking a glass of wine. I ate brewer's yeast tablets and drank gallons of liquid. I tried all the tricks. I've often said since, I would have swung from a trapeze by one toe if it would've helped.

Any mother who has pumped is likely to point out, emphatically, that a breast pump is not a baby!

Pumping can be distressing to the mother whose child does not yet receive her milk. But perhaps it is more difficult for the mother who pumps and believes strongly in breast-feeding, but seems to have almost no milk.

> After weeks of pumping every two to three hours, twenty-four hours a day, and getting only small amounts of milk, I was delivering my daily supply to the hospital when a nurse casually asked, "Is that all?"
>
> I wanted to scream, "Yes, that's all. I pump day and night for that milk and that's all!" I was very depressed at that innocent question.

HANDLING BREAST MILK

For specific instructions on collecting breast milk, consult the doctor or nurses who are caring for your baby. The following is a general outline of the most commonly recommended procedure for collecting and freezing breast milk:

1. Wash hands, breasts and all equipment to avoid contamination.
2. Sterilize any parts of the pump or collection containers that will come in contact with the milk. Some pumps require only washing with soap and hot water. Check the manufacturer's instructions.
3. On masking or freezer tape, write your baby's name, the date, the time when the milk was pumped, any medication you are taking and any other information the nursery requires. Instead of using tape, you may mark directly on some freezer containers with a permanent pen.
4. Pump and pour the milk into a disposable nurser bag or a sterile glass bottle. Check with the nursery about preferences on the type of container used. Ask your baby's doctor or nurse for advice on how much milk to put into each container.

    It may be helpful to separate each pumping into smaller batches before freezing. If several pumpings need to be combined to make up the necessary quantity of milk, use the layer method of freezing: chill freshly pumped milk and then pour it over frozen milk already in the container. Check with the hospital to be sure this method is acceptable.

5. If using disposable plastic nurser bags, close with a twist-tie or with a rubber band. When twist-ties are used, make sure the wire does not puncture the bag. Tape the ends of the wire and the edges of the bag with masking or freezer tape.

6. Freeze immediately.

Some of the milk's value, especially the immunities, is lost in freezing. If you pump at the hospital your baby can be fed fresh breast milk.

Fresh breast milk will keep for only twenty-four hours in the refrigerator. It may be kept frozen for up to two weeks in the freezer section of the refrigerator. If stored at a temperature of zero degrees Fahrenheit, breast milk may be kept for over three months.

When carrying breast milk to the hospital, it must be kept solidly frozen. Put containers of frozen milk in an ice chest with crushed ice or in some other suitable insulated container.

To thaw frozen breast milk, place the container of milk under running tap water, gradually increasing the water temperature from cold to hot. Shake the milk, as it will have separated. Once thawed, any unused milk should be discarded.

BREAST CARE

Because many mothers of premature infants have not had adequate time adequately to prepare their breasts for nursing and because pumping is harder on breasts and nipples than actual nursing, sore breasts and nipples are common. Soreness may occur either while pumping or during nursing.

The following suggestions have been found helpful by mothers who have encountered the problem. Check with the doctor before following any of these. Sometimes a combination of methods works best.

1. Wear a good nursing bra.
2. Do not use nursing pads at first and never use plastic-lined pads that restrict air circulation. Cloth diapers, cut into small squares and folded, or folded handkerchiefs will help absorb leaking milk. Breasts should be clean and dry before applying pads.
3. Allow air to circulate around the nipples by leaving the bra flaps down as much as possible. Sunlight can help heal sore nipples but limit exposure to avoid sunburn.
4. Avoid using soap on nipples; it can dry and crack them. Clean, warm water is sufficient for cleansing.
5. Use a light coat of breast cream, vegetable oil, or anhydrous lanolin (available at most pharmacies) to keep nipples from cracking. Nipples should be rinsed with water before pumping or nursing.
6. Place a 3-inch by 3-inch square of waxed paper, not plastic, over a liberal amount of breast cream on each nipple to prevent cracking or to promote healing of cracked or sore nipples. The waxed paper is worn under a nursing pad or bra and keeps the nipples moist and supple. This technique may not work for women with oily skin.
7. Touch the nipple with a piece of ice in a wet paper towel immediately before nursing. Cold will make the nipple erect so your baby can easily latch on, and ice will temporarily numb the nipple area. By the time numbness wears off, the discomfort of the initial latching on will have passed.
8. Change positions while nursing so that pressure will be put on different parts of the breast, thereby preventing unnecessary tenderness and engorgement.
9. Use a breast shield or rubber nipple over your own nipple. This technique should be used sparingly since your baby does need to become accustomed to the breast and nipples will eventually toughen up with use. Nipple soreness during the first weeks of nursing is common, but subsides in time.
10. Anticipate your baby's need to nurse. A frantically hungry baby will not be as gentle on the nipple. Short, frequent nursings are easier on nipples.
11. If you stop pumping or nursing, do so gradually to

avoid milk ducts becoming clogged or the breast becoming infected.

Engorgement and Clogged Milk Ducts

Most women become engorged to some extent when breast milk comes in during the first week after delivery. Initial engorgement usually goes away in a few days. However, it can still be very painful and may persist longer in some cases. Ice packs on the breasts can lessen the pain of initial engorgement. Some women feel more comfort from heat applications.

Clogged milk ducts may occur at any time during pumping or breast-feeding. While engorgement usually affects both breasts at the same time, a clogged milk duct is generally found in only one breast. The breast may feel lumpy or knotty and sore, and milk flow may be restricted.

To prevent having a clogged milk duct:

1. Be sure that each breast empties completely when pumping or nursing.
2. Be aware of schedule changes or of breasts that feel engorged.
3. Keep track of how long and how strongly your baby nurses on each side.
4. Massage the breasts while nursing and pump out remaining milk if the breasts still feel full.
5. Do not wear a tight bra since it may constrict the breasts and cause a duct to clog.
6. Change nursing positions.

For care of the breasts during engorgement or when there is a clogged milk duct:

1. Continue nursing or pumping on schedule.
2. Pump between nursing times or nurse more frequently.
3. Gently massage the breasts, paying special attention to lumpy areas, while pumping or nursing.
4. Apply a heating pad, moist compress or small hot water bottle.

5. Soak in a hot bath when allowed. A hot shower may be too painful or stimulating and could cause additional let-down of milk behind the clogged areas.

Engorgement or clogged milk ducts are usually temporary. If the condition persists, if there is redness of the breasts or if fever is present, contact the doctor.

BREAST-FEEDING A PREMIE

Breast-feeding in the hospital is sometimes difficult because of the lack of privacy or because of a mother's tension. Weighing the baby before and after feeding may be inhibiting. Many babies have become used to a bottle nipple; nursing from mother's breast is a completely new experience and may not be accepted right away. A small baby who has learned to suck from a bottle may have problems grasping and sucking a large and unfamiliarly shaped nipple and areola.

If your baby will not nurse or nurses poorly, do not be discouraged. Your baby may do better once home. Just relax and enjoy this close physical contact with your baby.

Your baby may need to rest occasionally, as sucking from the breast is tiring to a premature infant. Watch for an overactive let-down reflex when milk comes out too fast, causing baby to choke. To compensate for milk coming too quickly, place the first two fingers of your free hand in a V around your nipple and gently compress to restrict the flow of milk. You can then regulate the milk flow as baby's needs change. If your baby fusses because milk is not coming quickly enough, gently massage the breast as though hand expressing while nursing to increase the milk flow. Also, make sure that the breast is not completely covering baby's nose and interfering with breathing.

Changing from a bottle to breast after baby comes home can bring new problems. If you are having difficulty making the switch, here are some ideas that may help. Check with your baby's doctor before following any of these suggestions:

1. If your baby shows little interest in sucking, put a dab of light Karo syrup under your nipples. The taste may encourage sucking. Do not use honey, since it can cause infant botulism in babies under one year of age.
2. Sometimes dipping a long cotton swab in water and tickling the roof of a baby's mouth may encourage sucking. This cannot be done with babies who have respiratory problems or who are on respirators. In individual cases, a special technique that is effective might be found. One mother discovered that stroking a spot behind her child's ear would stimulate the baby's sucking reflex.
3. Try to stimulate let-down or hand express some milk before putting baby to the breast. The smell and taste of your milk may encourage sucking.
4. When having to supplement with a bottle, use either a Nuk or Playtex nipple instead of the standard type.
5. If your baby is having a hard time grasping the nipple, try inserting more of it into the mouth. Or try touching ice to the nipple to make it more erect.
6. Use a spoon, eyedropper or syringe for supplemental feedings to avoid baby's becoming dependent on a bottle nipple.
7. Change positions while nursing.
8. If possible, use breast milk obtained by pumping for supplemental feedings.
9. Use a breast shield or premie nipple over your own nipple, but do so sparingly.
10. Try the Lact-Aid nursing supplementer, (fig. 12)
11. Have a friend or relative at home give your baby any necessary supplemental bottle while you pump out milk remaining in your breasts.
12. Seek help and support from your doctor, nurse, relatives, a nursing mother or support group.

It may take considerable time and determination to gradually change over to a totally breast-fed baby. Get to know your baby's feeding preferences to decide what is best for both of you.

The problem is basically one of readjustment by the infant.

Occasionally the infant rejects all efforts at breast-feeding. In this case, the mother may choose to switch to formula altogether or to continue pumping and offer breast milk in a bottle.

First Attempts at Nursing

While the infant is hospitalized, a clinical interest is taken in the amount of milk consumed at each feeding. It can be disconcerting to a nursing mother to have her infant whisked away to the scales before the feeding can be labeled a success or a failure. In the eyes of the mother, the closeness with her baby makes the venture a success. In the eyes of the nurses and doctors responsible for the child's care, no appreciable weight gain makes the venture a failure and may prompt a decision to delay further attempts at breast-feeding. One mother, who had pumped for seventy-five days before nursing, tells of her first breast-feeding experience and the tension that the matter of weight gain can add to the situation:

> I left home hurriedly; I couldn't get to the hospital fast enough. When I got there, the nurse asked me if I was going to try to breast-feed Mindy. I looked at her in puzzlement and said, "Yes." I thought, "What did she mean—try to breast-feed?"
>
> The nurse then took Mindy and removed her hat and blankets and weighed her. Then she handed Mindy to me, pointed to the room and told me she would bring a washrag in so that I could wipe off my breasts. She brought the washrag in and told me I would have ten minutes to try to breast-feed Mindy. There it was again, "try."
>
> I was very excited when she left because this was the first time I was ever totally alone with my baby. Yet I was nervous, too. I had never breast-fed a baby before, and now I was supposed to do it on my own.
>
> "Mindy, I don't really know what I'm doing. I sure hope you can help me." I held her close to me, and she looked up at me as if to say, "Mom, what am I supposed to do?" I had thought together we would manage. I was completely wrong.

> She groped around trying very hard to get a hold on
> my nipple without much luck. I think she really sensed
> how important this was to me because she didn't cry or
> fuss, she just kept trying.
>
> The nurse came in and said that we didn't want to tire
> Mindy out so she took Mindy and put her on the scales.
> It registered that she had gained 10 cc. I was proud to
> think that for my and her first try, we were able to get
> her to drink 10 cc. I had whispered to her before we went
> to weigh, "Come on, Mindy, weigh a lot more. Show
> those nurses that we can do it."
>
> The next try at breast-feeding came the next day. We
> were completely unsuccessful. She weighed no differ-
> ently. So I told her that was okay; when we got home,
> things would be different. I would be more relaxed and
> she would be, too.

Parents should consider the special needs of their child. Most
premies need extra iron. Some also need additional vitamins or
minerals.

In addition to these problems, communication can break down
between the medical staff and a mother who wants to breast-
feed.

> The doctor told me that formula had been the game
> plan for Bonni all along. Well, simply put, I exploded! If
> that had been the game plan all along, then I wanted to
> play too. We felt that it was only fair that we be in-
> formed about every new change in Bonni's condition
> and care.
>
> Soon we realized the extremely delicate balance a 670-
> gram baby's system is in and how carefully the doctors
> must plan each new step forward to protect the child's
> life.

Rarely, a parent may be able to influence medical decisions
regarding the infant's feeding. A mother whose son's "last days"
in the hospital "stretched into weeks" because of his inability to
bottle-feed without choking, falling asleep or having episodes of
bradycardia defends the importance of having asserted her beliefs:

I also believed that Jonah should be fed on demand, but his method of demand was not initially understood. He was awakened every three hours for a feeding. The nurses reported that he rarely woke up crying to be fed.

It seemed difficult for Jonah to make the necessary association between being hungry and sucking. He was never really given the chance to experience the discomfort of hunger. I mentioned this to his primary nurse. She agreed, and with the doctor's approval, initiated a demand feeding schedule.

Once this was begun, Jonah slept seven hours at a stretch. Within two days of demand feeding, he started to lose weight. Weight loss was seen as a setback, but I still believed Jonah would have to feel hunger to demand food, and that what was really necessary for us to learn was his method of communicating hunger.

After speaking with two mothers who had premature babies, I realized that instead of crying for food, he might be signaling his hunger by bodily movements. There was the possibility that six weeks on a respirator and with feeding tubes in his throat had irritated him so much that crying was much too painful.

I asked to take a more aggressive role and received permission to move him into a separate room where I could stay with him around the clock. I wanted to be able to nurse him in response to his signals of hunger. It worked.

Within three days, he was nursing sufficiently well and he began to put on weight. The doctor was so pleased with Jonah's progress that I was given permission the following day to bring him home.

SWITCHING FROM BOTTLE TO BREAST AT HOME

After the baby comes home, a mother who wants to nurse can find herself feeling very alone when faced with an infant who doesn't suck well. One mother, whose daughter came home weighing 3 pounds 10 ounces, ran the gamut of solutions to this problem: crosscut premie nipples, Nuk r nipples, a premie nipple used as a breast shield, different nursing positions, forcing more of her own nipple into her daughter's mouth, hand expressing milk into her daughter's mouth, putting Karo syrup under her nipple, putting an eyedropperful of milk into her daughter's mouth while nursing, and spoon-feeding the supplemental feedings instead of giving a bottle. The daughter held out, knowing that she would eventually receive a bottle.

With a strict reminder that the baby was not to go more than four hours without milk, the pediatrician gave permission to eliminate bottle-feedings altogether.

> If the ear syringe used as an emergency feeding measure hadn't worked, I probably would have quit. I gave myself, or should I say her, two more days, and if she hadn't taken to the breast after that I would have given up willingly, knowing that I had done and tried everything I knew. I am glad I didn't have to make that decision.
>
> When she cried, I cried but we finally made it. Yes, I think it was worth it.

Another problem is the sleepy baby. Premies tire easily. It is common for a baby to fall asleep in the middle of a feeding. Waking the baby may not be an adequate solution, especially if the infant falls asleep several times during a feeding.

In the hospital, any baby who does not gain weight is a major concern. If a hospitalized premie tires repeatedly while nursing, the nursery staff may tell the mother to stop breast-feeding, and feed the baby by gavage tube or bottle. At home, if the baby's weight gain is stable and the problem is merely one of fatigue, the mother may find that the baby makes up for sleeping at feedings by eating more frequently or by accepting a supplemental bottle between feedings. Either situation can be exhausting for mother, and sometimes father, too!

> After two weeks at home, Jennifer weighed 5½ pounds and the doctor said she was strong enough to nurse. But her mouth was still so small and she tired so easily that our routine for the next two weeks was that she would nurse a few minutes until she became tired and/or too frustrated; then I would pump while Eddie fed her with

the premie nipple and bottle. Needless to say, we were all frustrated and exhausted.

After two weeks of this, my doctor suggested that she was strong enough to drop the bottle-feedings completely. The first two days she screamed out of hunger and frustration as she was really having to work so much harder. But it worked, and she was finally totally breast-fed.

Only a healthy baby, with the permission of the pediatrician, can be made to work for feedings in this manner. A hospitalized premie cannot be allowed to become exhausted from sucking because of the calorie loss involved.

Supplementing

Supplemental feedings are common, if not essential, for many premies. The totally breast-fed premature baby is in the minority. One pro-nursing mother described her situation:

Zachary seemed always hungry. We'd attempted to nurse on demand his first week home, with no supplementing or pumping. However, much to my horror, he lost 3 ounces. I was sure my pediatrician would put him back in the hospital. I blamed myself for starving Zachary and endangering his health. After that, I wasn't as opposed to supplementing with formula as I had been.

One side benefit of supplementing was that I could nurse until the formula was warmed. By then, my milk was gone and he was content to take his bottle more slowly, which meant that he did not choke so often.

Occasionally, breast milk is implicated in the development of "breast-milk" jaundice. A hormone in the mother's milk interferes with the action of an enzyme in the baby's liver. In some cases, treatment is to withhold breast milk for several days, during which time the mother can pump to maintain her supply.

Drying Up

When it is time to stop breast-feeding, many women have difficulty drying up their milk supply. Such difficulty may occur either with gradual weaning or with a sudden halt to nursing necessitated by the health of mother or infant. Drying up seems to take longer after each subsequent breast-fed child and can take as long as six months.

For some women, the breasts may leak or swell and become painfully engorged. When this happens, ice packs or heat may alleviate pain. Liquid intake should be restricted and nipple stimulation avoided. The doctor should be notified if any signs of infection such as fever, hard lumps or redness are present.

If the breasts become too uncomfortable or if the milk supply does not seem to be diminishing, check with the doctor for further advice.

A mother who was told to dry up as a result of her daughter's lactose intolerance said:

> When the time for Monica's release from the hospital came nearer, my milk came in again. I woke up one morning to find that I had flooded the bed with my milk. This can be an unnerving experience, especially if you had intended to nurse, because your body seems to want to continue in an unbroken chain of mothering abilities, even if your mind knows that there are some things you can't do. The nurses reassured me that stresses can cause many changes in milk supply that are absolutely normal.

A SHOULDER TO LEAN ON

Some mothers have a strong inner determination to nurse and few problems with milk supply. Such mothers are able to pump for a long period of time without much apparent need for encouragement from others. These women are rare!

At the very least, a mother who chooses to pump and attempt nursing a premature infant needs support and encouragement from her husband.

One woman's husband who was exceptionally supportive after

their first son was born expressed his "secret doubts" about her pumping days several years later. He told her that he even had wondered "why she didn't want to get milk for their baby," at a time when her milk supply was virtually nonexistent. She was grateful for his support during those hard times, but she was also glad, after her shock, that he had shared his thoughts with her later.

> Just telling a father to be encouraging and supportive isn't enough. He often rents a breast pump for his wife while she is still in the hospital. When the pump is received, he usually gets both verbal and written instructions on how to stimulate a milk supply. Thus, he may get a 1-2-3 idea of pumping. Fathers may think that just following the directions and suggestions will automatically produce a milk supply.
>
> Father must understand the relationship of emotional stress to the mother's ability to produce milk. If she is having difficulty and is trying to pump, she is probably doing all that is humanly possible. Whatever the amount she produces, the effort and stress of pumping make the results enough.

Beyond a father's support, a mother needs, at the minimum, an acceptance of her efforts by her family and the medical staff caring for her and her infant.

> The intensive care nursery nurses were wonderful and offered constant encouragement. Their remarks would really boost my morale. In the early stages when I was getting so little milk, they explained how it was more than enough for one feeding and how beneficial breast milk was for my baby. Later they oohed and aahed at my production when I pumped at the hospital and reminded me to save the excess for Sara when she got home. It was great to hear them talk about her coming home!
>
> My milk supply dropped as the big day drew near, but again the nurses reassured me that it was not unusual and would pick up again once Sara was home to nurse all the time.

Support can also come from unexpected sources.

> We met another couple whose premature son was next
> to Zachary in ICU. Soon we were friends and comrades
> in a common struggle. We'd meet at visitation hour, and
> out in the hall, surrounded by a crowd of other worried
> families, we exchanged concerns and information on
> how to pump breast milk.
>
> On one visit, this couple told how they had discovered
> that if Bruce gently twisted, turned or rubbed one nipple
> while Nila pumped the other breast, then the stimulation
> would help prepare the other breast for pumping. Bruce
> then began to demonstrate the technique in the air.
>
> Chet and I watched and listened attentively. We were
> all so deadly serious that it was funny. Here we were in
> a crowd—two couples, newly met—and we were discuss-
> ing nipple stimulation. All modesty disappears in such
> emergency situations. They had valuable information,
> and we wanted it!
>
> Chet and Bruce would discuss how much breast milk
> we'd produced at the last pumping as if they were com-
> paring gasoline mileage.

Often, the mother of a premie needs as much support in deciding not to continue to pump as she needed when she first chose
to do so. A mother who discontinues pumping may feel that she
has wasted her time or that she has "failed" at breast-feeding.
Once the initial disappointment is faced, however, many mothers feel relieved. They begin to concentrate on other ways of
nurturing their baby. One of the most important support systems
a pumping or nursing mother can have is that of other mothers
who have encountered similar difficulties.

A GOOD MOTHER IS WHAT COUNTS

If there is any word that should not be used in a discussion of
breast-feeding, it is "failure." A mother who does not have a large
milk supply is not a "failure." A mother whose infant takes little
milk at the first nursing encounter is not a "failure." A mother

who has to dry up because her child cannot tolerate milk is not a "failure."

> I bottle-fed Traleena, my first child. Mindy, my premie, I breast-fed. I enjoyed breast-feeding, but I would not have changed anything about my bottle-feeding experience either. I feel that I was just as close to each of my daughters.
>
> A good mother is what counts. We were fortunate to have had a premature baby survive to eat. Loving the baby is what matters—not how the baby is fed.

Chapter 9

LOOKING INTO THE FUTURE

Milestones in the development of a premie take on delightful significance. Each time these babies roll over, grasp toys, crawl, walk or talk, they reaffirm that they are alive. Some of these children are ones that doctors warned parents would probably never walk or talk, or even live.

> At five years of age, Monica's existence can still cause friends and acquaintances to shake their heads and say, "Can you believe?" "I can remember when I thought that tadpole would never make it!" "Do you realize how healthy she is?"
>
> Despite intestinal surgery when she weighed 2 pounds and 3 ounces, she is (over) active and a charmer!
>
> Sometimes it gives me a special warmth in my heart of hearts to know that my child can give another human being a sense of hope.

NAGGING FEARS

Current statistics indicate that of the estimated 300,000 infants who are born prematurely each year in the United States, 90 percent live. Some of those who live are more likely to have physical, emotional or mental disabilities. But which ones?

A statistical survey by Parents of Prematures, Houston, asked parents of premature infants what most concerned them about their children in the first years of of life. Their first responses were, overwhelmingly, about specific illnesses or problems; second about development and how it would affect their children's future. (See page 000 for a summary of the survey.)

When a parent asks, "Will my child have permanent problems?" doctors often are unable to give a definite answer. The procedures used to save a baby may be so new that any long-term consequences of treatment are unknown. The parents are left in emotional turmoil: They are overjoyed that their child has survived, but they live with nagging fears that their child may never outgrow certain problems or that there may be future difficulties ahead.

It is normal for parents to continue to react to a premature birth for several months, even years, after the event.

> The most convincing evidence of my continued emotional distress during Zachary's first year was my uncontrollable reaction to anything concerning pregnancy or new babies. Television commercials depicting smiling mothers with new babies or programs that showed a perfect pregnancy would reduce me to tears.
>
> It sounds ridiculous to have been so emotional, but I believe it was part of my "mourning process." I was mourning the loss of a normal pregnancy, a normal coming home, and a normal beginning with our baby.
>
> Taking Zachary home from the hospital didn't automatically end the emotional stress I'd been under. I defused slowly. The bouts of crying were just steam valves, relieving some of the self-contained pressures.

Parents with legitimate concerns about the development of their child know that there are many steps between the initial worry and finally obtaining help.

> Mindy was born three months early. I knew that developmentally she would not be doing things a child of her birth age would do. I accepted that fact and learned to shrug off remarks people made, like "You mean at twelve months she's not crawling yet? She should be walking!"
>
> I did realize that Mindy was slower than I thought she should be. I kept telling the doctor that I thought she should go to a developmental center to be evaluated. I wanted to know if there was something we could do to help her catch up. For four months this went on. Her doctor would tell me, "Now, remember she was three months early and that would put her three months behind her age." Like I was going to forget!
>
> I needed support. I talked to two mothers in Parents of Prematures [whose children had been through a developmental center in Houston]. They gave me the support and encouragement I needed to forcefully express my concerns to the physician.
>
> When Mindy was fourteen months old, I told the doctor that I and my husband were concerned about her development. She was not walking, pulling up, crawling or standing on her feet. I told him I had seen newborns stand on their feet as a reflex better than my daughter did. The doctor then said, "Yes, we really need to do something about that." I'm still convinced that he finally decided to because I said my husband was concerned.

Soon after talking to her daughter's doctor, this mother contacted the city health department. A therapist evaluated Mindy at home and suggested that she have physical and speech therapy at the city clinic. She also instructed the mother how to do therapy at home. There was no charge for this service.

Later, Mindy was tested at the developmental center and the professionals there approved of the regimen of care she was receiving. At age three, Mindy has caught up; she is walking, talking and no longer requires therapy.

Other prematurely born children show no particular susceptibility to illnesses or signs of significant developmental delays in
their first years of life. Parents of these children understand how
fortunate they and their children are. David's mother summed
up the thoughts of many parents:

> Although David has never been sick with anything other
> than a virus, it still took us a good year to relax and not
> worry about "what could possibly happen." Now he is
> nineteen months old and catching up beautifully. How
> can we help but feel blessed?

DEVELOPMENT

It is true that prematurity is often associated with serious medical problems like cerebral palsy, mental retardation, epilepsy and
autism; with handicaps like blindness, deafness and cleft palate;
and with other less serious problems such as hyperactivity or
learning disabilities. It has been argued that the increasing ability
to save premature infants would result in an increased number
of permanently handicapped children. However, a recent study
disputes this argument. It currently appears that much of the
residual "damage" found in children who were born too early
relates to various types of learning disabilities. Even so, it is still
too early to tell if these learning difficulties are long-term or
temporary. (McCleary, Elliot H., *New Miracles of Childbirth:
How Modern Medical Miracles Are Making Childbearing Safer
and Easier*)

Parents should be cautious when they read or hear anything
concerning the mental or physical development of premies. It is
often impossible for parents to assess the validity of information
on their own, due to rapid advances in neonatology. Statistics in
medical textbooks become quickly outdated. The best source of
medical information is the doctor caring for the child.

What can generally be said about the development of premies,
whether or not they had serious problems at birth, is that they
often have difficulty with neurologic integration. Their biological
timetable for integrating visual, auditory and motor abilities may

not be matched to the timetable generally followed by babies born at term. As a result, premature infants are easily distracted; they may not be able to shut out stimuli sufficiently. Due to all of these factors, premies may tire easily. Unfortunately for their parents, premature children are as likely to become "unglued" when fatigued as they are likely to act sleepy. (Tiffany Martini Field, ed., *Infants Born at Risk: Behavior and Development*) These problems of integration can last long past infancy.

What are the implications of these problems in parenting premature children? One mother responded:

> It takes patience, patience and sometimes more patience than I have to keep her on track. She's not hyperactive in the clinical sense, but she's so active! I can remember having to lie down with her at nap time and put my arm around her just to get her to stop!

Many parents whose premature infants survive with little or no obvious difficulties still must cope with active, strong-willed or frustrated children who develop according to their own individual timetable. Patience and observation are needed to make the best assessment of such a child's needs. Karen's story is typical:

> Karen's motor development seemed slow. She was crawling, pulling herself into a sitting position and standing by eleven months of age—but she learned to do all of those things in that one month. Before then, she was a frustrated and angry child. I believe that she was mentally ready to do these things for months, but was physically unable to do them. If I laid her on the floor she would have a temper tantrum; she was probably tired of looking at the floor or ceiling!
>
> To keep her happy, I carried her everywhere for almost a full year. I didn't mind, though, as I felt it was one way to make up for the lost time in utero. Also, she was light as a feather—she weighed 14 pounds at one year— and being held kept her contented.
>
> Now at nearly five years of age, she is enjoying her gymnastics class and ballet. She always has a big grin on her face and has enough energy for two children.

As stated in a chapter one, it is impossible to judge a premie's development strictly by "adjusted age." It is also impossible to say definitely that by a certain age (those usually mentioned are age two or three or by school age) a child who was born prematurely will be completely caught up with developmental norms.

Occasionally, developmental problems continue to exist for a number of years. Most are not life-threatening but they do affect a family in many ways. One mother told this story about her eight-year-old son:

> He has learning disabilities—short attention span, poor auditory and visual memory. His main area of disturbance occurs in a classroom situation, where the increased stimulus of twenty-six children and the need to follow directions and cope with independent work periods leads to hyperactivity and a discipline problem. This led to a decrease in motivation and good attitude. On a 1–3 ratio he functioned well but [in] a classroom—not a chance. He said, "I don't know why I get in so much trouble all the time. I don't mean to."
>
> A local pediatrician who deals with learning-disabled children put him on [medication]. The result was marvelous . . . now he can receive, process and return information. His attitude about school has improved greatly, as have all aspects of his school work and behavior. This medication doesn't work for all [children], but . . . in combination with a thirty-minute-per-day special education program, all is going well for him now.

Premies with handicaps or severe medical problems have special problems of development.

> Our daughter's cerebral palsy (CP) was not evident at birth. The first months we looked with optimism towards normalcy. However, when Angela was nine months of age, we became suspicious of her developmental lags. But it wasn't until she was one year old that we could get medical professionals to discuss our fears with us.
>
> The doctors were apprehensive about making an early diagnosis of such a severe disability as CP for fear that labeling would set limits on our expectations and those of

the medical field, society and Angela.

Finally, a mother in a parents of prematures group listened to my fears and suggested several books I could read. One book written for parents that really helped us was *Handling the Young Cerebral Palsied Child at Home* by Nancie R. Finnie (New York: Dutton-Sunrise, Inc., 1974).

At age fifteen months, Angela was just beginning to roll over—she couldn't sit or balance. It was then we were given the first medical diagnosis. The doctors still wouldn't use the term CP although we, her parents, were already using it. They were still calling it "developmental lag" or "disability."

We resented it. We felt they were trying to sugarcoat a very serious problem. No one would suggest we take Angela to a developmental center, so we had to insist that our pediatrician refer her.

At that time, we contacted the developmental center and we also called the CP center. Angela started physical, occupational and speech therapy at fifteen months. We felt she should have started at six months.

When CP was finally diagnosed, we felt a sense of disbelief and shock that normalcy would never be possible. But we also felt relief that at least we knew where we were and what avenues we could take toward hope and progress.

Angela is now four years old. Her physical abilities remain at the age level of a nine- to twelve-month old. Her gross motor abilities are limited to floor creeping and supported sitting. Her social and intellectual skills and speech are appropriate for her age. She is a self-secure and enthusiastic child who feels few limitations.

We're very proud of her! Her zest for life and people have made us much more aware of people's abilities rather than their disabilities. We take no ability for granted.

MAKING COMPARISONS

Most parents realize their child should not be compared to any other child. A term baby who does not sit up until eleven months of age might be considered "slow." A premature infant who was three months early and does not sit up until eleven months may be considered perfectly normal. That premature child cannot even be compared to another premie who was three months early and who sat up unsupported at eight months.

Intellectually, parents know that their children are unique. But the continual state of awareness needed to watch carefully the progress of premies results in constant comparisons.

Evaluation of one child's development versus another's is almost inevitable in parent support groups, no matter how much the individuality of each child is emphasized and reemphasized. While such comparisons may cause some concern, parent support groups also offer an atmosphere of camaraderie, where positive comments on a baby's progress come from parents who know, who have watched their own premie, and perhaps others in the group, grow and develop.

Another important point to remember is that everything premies do or do not do is not necessarily a result of their prematurity.

> Every baby has a pace of his own. In addition to your child's prematurity, it is important to remember that your child's personality will influence his style and rate of development in all areas . . . large muscle, small muscle, social and so forth.
>
> In *Infants and Mothers* (New York: Delacorte Press, 1969), Dr. T. Berry Brazelton discusses three different types of babies—active, average and quiet—demonstrating how broad the spectrum of normal development can be.
>
> Some babies are simply content to lie back and let life go on around them . . . observing but not actively participating. Is this baby "slow" or merely displaying a more passive personality?

The mother who made this comment did so with another mother in mind:

> She had four term boys and then a little girl born prematurely. I met her when the baby was ten months old and she was beginning to be very concerned that her daughter was not developing as her sons had.
>
> After discussing this with her pediatrician, she took the child to the developmental center, where the child was further observed and evaluated. It was decided that the baby had a very passive personality. The mother had been familiar only with busy, active babies.
>
> Today this little girl is seventeen months old and remains very docile and quiet. But the mother now sees her daughter as an individual different from her other children.

Questions of size, rate of growth, weight gain, physical coordination, mental development and the need for discipline are constant grounds for comparison. All parents, not only parents of premies, are concerned about their child's development and behavior.

THE NEW STATISTICS

In the 1970s, parents were confronted by such statements as: "Parents of prematures are prime candidates to be child abusers." "Premature children are always so immature." "Premature children do not respond well to affection."

The statements and statistics regarding the consequences of prematurity have been overwhelmingly negative. They have led many a parent to wonder, "Will I abuse my child? Will my child always be emotionally scarred?"

However, most of the children mentioned in this book are part of a new set of statistics. They were not totally separated from their parents in the early days of their lives. Perhaps this change in policy will invalidate the statements and improve the statistics —we hope so.

BECOMING A FAMILY

Time is needed to integrate any new baby into a family. For parents of premies, the baby's needs during their initial years of life must be balanced with the needs of the rest of the family.

Where the difficulties the child encounters are not severe or where parents are dealing with their first child, the baby's development may not seem unusual. This is especially true if the child's difficulties are outgrown in time.

> Johanna and Suzanne were born twelve weeks early weighing 2 pounds and 2 ounces each. I worried about their development, but their pediatrician continually encouraged us that they would be fine. That first year, I just couldn't believe that we could have such small twins and have them both come out perfectly healthy and normal.
>
> They walked at sixteen months and were speaking sentences by the age of two. They're 3½ years old now and they've never had any developmental problems. They're small, the size of two-year-olds, and that sometimes keeps them from doing things larger children can. For instance, they couldn't ride a tricycle until they were older, not because they couldn't pedal, but because they couldn't reach the pedals.
>
> I would tell parents of premies not to set goals and expectations based on developmental norms; then they won't be disappointed or frustrated.

As outlooks for premies continue to improve, more and more parents find that eventually their problems in rearing their child are simply problems of parenting.

However, one particular worry for parents of premature infants is their concern that "something else is going to happen." In this instance, it is true that a little learning is a dangerous thing. Parents may hear that a particular handicap or health problem is more commonly found among children who were born prematurely. Parents do need to be aware that problems can arise but such awareness should never be confused with overanxious watching.

Let them explore, get their knocks and learn by doing. Hopefully they'll surprise you, and you'll find that all your anxiety was groundless . . . . If you let them sense that you're afraid something may be wrong with them, they just may live up to your expectations.

In the course of growing up, these children sometimes must be rehospitalized, or they may experience a series of minor problems or seem especially susceptible to childhood illnesses. They may also exhibit puzzling signs of nonspecific developmental problems.

Each time a new health or developmental problem arises, fears lingering in parents' minds and old feelings may be reawakened.

We can say that the helpless feeling we now have about Jennie's slow development has been the hardest cross to bear. We have, however, accepted the possibility that Jennie may be handicapped even in her adulthood and know that we will do all possible to help her reach as normal a level of functioning as she can, with God's help.

We are thankful that our precious daughter is alive and in good health and realize that other parents of prematures have not been so fortunate.

For some parents and their children, legitimate concerns about health and prematurity extend past the first years into the future.

One cold winter night when Ryan was eighteen months old, he awoke at 3 a.m. with croup. I had never heard a child with croup and thought he had developed an instant pneumonia, which we had been warned could happen. We rushed him to the emergency room of the closest hospital. The doctor on call read his chest X rays and saw the scar tissue but was unsure of its origin. The next morning, our pediatrician looked at the X rays and immediately recognized them as old scars from the respirator, not pneumonia. My mind was at ease, but for those few hours I was fearing the worst.

Then at twenty-two months, Ryan choked on a few

tiny bites of an apple. My whacking him on the back and
putting my finger down his throat were to no avail, and
the paramedics had to be called. We were able to revive
him using first-aid techniques; however, the paramedic
wanted to check him out thoroughly.

After listening through his stethoscope, he asked,
"What kind of chronic illness does your child have?" I
related Ryan's history of respiratory problems and explained that his lungs still sound "like two pieces of sand-
paper rubbing against each other." Still he insisted we go
to the hospital for a chest X ray and thorough checkup.
I had our personal pediatrician again check the X ray for
the familiar scar tissue still present.

I realize that this is only the beginning. Since we are
moving 1,500 miles from here this month, I foresee a
recurrence of these scenes many, many times. The presence of this scar tissue is also something my son will need
to be aware of since it will show up on X rays even as an
adult.

When children have serious problems, parents may feel a blow
to their self-esteem or they may perceive themselves, their families and their babies in a new and different way.

Our family, with the Lord's help, has come through this
experience with peace. My baby has brought so much
love.

I feel my biggest problem is me—I want to protect her
too much and do too much for her.

One mother, who was told with her husband "not to form an
attachment to your daughter because she is probably going to
die," indicates the kinds of feelings parents can have even after
a number of years:

It is still—she is now 8½ years old—difficult to assess the
repercussions of her prematurity on her subsequent
growth and development. From the moment of her
birth, she has always been on her own timetable which,
more often than not, did not jibe with that of her peers.

She did not, as the hospital pediatrician told us, catch

up after two to 2½ years. Not only did this cause considerable difficulty when she was an infant and toddler when so much revolves around "size," but also later on when she entered school and teachers tried to push her before she was ready.

Eventually, hopefully, the premature infant will become a child whose demands can be put into perspective and who can be seen as a "constant joy" rather than a cause for worry.

THE ONCE AND FUTURE CHILD

Even today it is almost impossible to predict the future for any premature baby.

Some parents live with a lifelong responsibility of caring for a handicapped child because of problems resulting from prematurity. Others are able to put their child's prematurity aside after a few years and simply become parents raising a child.

The children mentioned in stories throughout this book are like children everywhere and yet they are special, too. They are, above all else, themselves.

At age four, Michael has been in preschool for two years. He is now enjoying gymnastics and is learning to swim.

He finally sleeps through the night! During the daytime, he does his share of family chores and is fascinated by our home computer. (He can type in commands and set up and play some of the computer games.)

He has a good memory for stories, songs and sequential tasks. He loves to take his toys apart and put them together again!

It has been four years since Trey was born and had RDS and other complications of his prematurity. It is especially difficult for me to realize that when I hear his voice loud and clear—over the television, the voices of other people, even my husband's race car motor!

He has had no eye problems or any apparent lasting effects from the RDS he had at birth.

He is an assertive little boy, always full of questions and observant of the minutest details.

Although Ryan's X rays still show some scars from the respirator, his lung capacity has greatly improved. Now four years old, he is even swimming!
He enjoyed nursery school last year and next year will begin preschool. His preschool physical showed him caught up in all areas of development.

The strong will to live that Susan showed at birth is still present, three years later. Despite being headstrong, she is also a friendly, loving child.
Strangers are drawn to her sweet smile and mischievous grin, her big beautiful blue eyes and long eyelashes. They are amazed too that this small little girl speaks so clearly and says things that seem beyond her years.
Next year, she begins preschool. Whenever I look at her doll-size coming-home outfit and that first photograph of her, I can hardly believe she was ever that small or that I was so fearful of losing her. It's like the whole experience was a dream—not bad, not good—just a dream.

Charlie is another "special child" who, at age three, has been hospitalized at least twice a year with respiratory problems. His parents say that his "inhalation therapy machine is as familiar as his trucks and trains." Charlie enjoys doing all the things any normal child would enjoy.
After beginning nursery school and finally being out of a two-year isolation from other children, another problem surfaced:

We thought we had it all licked. One morning I got a call at work from Charlie's school. They informed me that they were on the way to the hospital with him. It seemed that he had had some sort of seizure and was unconscious. That was the first time anything had ever happened without me being there. I couldn't get much information from the school so I rushed to the hospital. I could not believe this was happening! I arrived to find a child that was still having seizure activity. I had never

seen him do anything like that before. He was so gray.
His eyes were open but . . . he responded to nothing. I
thought he was dying. This lasted about five hours. All of
a sudden he snapped out of it. He had been given a
massive dose of phenobarbitol, but at least he could see
me and respond to me.

After many tests and four more seizures, his parents were told
that the seizures were probably a result of hypoxia, lack of oxygen, at birth. The large amount of medication Charlie must take
each day has become a part of his family's daily routine. But his
parents add:

We will endure this latest problem. We have endured
much more than we ever thought we could. I suspect we
can take much more. Charlie's smile and twinkling eyes
can make you forget all the pain and sorrow.

Editor's note: Charlie has been accepted by his school
district for their early childhood program.

Zachary's parents have raised their "whirlwind" for five years
now. His mother offered these words:

The premature baby I've written about doesn't exist anymore. In that baby's place is a bright, healthy five-year-
old boy. He has a head full of hair. His legs are long and
strong, and he's tall for his age.
    Zachary loves to rough and tumble with his daddy and
be a daredevil by leaping off tables and beds. He's curious
and independent. He likes to draw, to build cities out of
blocks and to dig outside in the sand.
    Zachary is reading books on a third-grade level and
shows promise of being a gifted learner. He's loving,
mischievous and wonderful. His most serious ailments in
five years have been occasional colds. He's a regular,
normal, very loved boy.
    The parents that brought home that premature baby
don't exist anymore either. In their place are parents that
have been strengthened and relieved of the burden of
fears brought home with the baby.

The memories we have of Zachary's birth, hospitalization and first year have been tempered with experience, perspective and time. When we talk about that past, it is with a sense of sadness, but a sadness we can now bear. It's much like remembering someone you loved who has died. The hurt is eased by the passage of time.

DEVELOPMENTAL CENTERS

The first years of a premature baby's life are critical ones for the child's future. During this time, a baby's developmental progress as well as health should be checked periodically. Routine follow-up should include evaluation of the child's feeding and sleeping patterns; motor, mental, social and emotional development; vision and hearing; and neurological and physical development.

The goal of early assessment is not to predict the future but to discover the child's strengths and weaknesses. With this knowledge, a plan for comprehensive medical and developmental evaluation and treatment can be formulated. Early treatment may help some children overcome problems more quickly and easily.

Traditionally, pediatricians have worked with parents to assess a child's health and development. However, babies born at risk or those with established developmental delays or handicaps are now often referred by their pediatrician to other medical or developmental specialists or to developmental centers.

Developmental centers exist in most large cities in the United States. They are generally located at hospitals, universities, medical schools, research centers or private clinics. A few are operated by local or county government agencies. Many cities, unfortunately, do not have such centers, and there is no single reliable source of information for parents regarding resources that are available for children at developmental risk.

Pediatricians or pediatric neurologists usually can advise parents on what services are available on local and state levels. The child's pediatrician is in a good position to act as the coordinator of the child's assessment and treatment, including therapy, even when referrals to professionals who practice at different locations is necessary. Parents may wish to ask the neonatologists who cared for their child or the delivering obstetrician for the names of pediatricians in their community who have reputations for being interested in the care of children who may have developmental problems.

If a child is referred to a developmental center, parents will be asked to provide information and to work with their child as needed between visits to the center. At most centers, a team of professionals assesses the child's abilities and needs. A developmental center team may include the following professionals:

- Developmental pediatrician and/or pediatric neurologist
- Psychiatrist or psychologist
- Child developmentalist and/or early childhood education specialist
- Physical therapist
- Speech and language therapist
- Nurses
- Social workers

Other specialists, such as orthopedic surgeons, ophthalmologists and audiometricians, are available for consultation if needed. Social workers, visiting home nurses or parent educators often act as liaisons between the specialists and the parents.

Preferably, the professional team is located in one place so that both the child and the parents can become comfortable in a familiar setting and have a complete understanding of the child's status and treatment.

Ultimately, it is the parents and day-to-day experiences that will have the strongest and most enduring impact on the child's development. Any program of treatment and therapy should take into consideration the knowledge, feeling and skills of the child's parents.

FAMOUS PREMATURE BABIES

In making comparisons, parents may find it encouraging to remember this list of famous premies from the past and present:

Isaac Newton
Charles Robert Darwin
Winston Churchill
Voltaire
Jean Jacques Rousseau
Victor Hugo
Napoleon Bonaparte
Ex-King Farouk of Egypt
Willie Shoemaker
Joey Bishop
Renoir
Albert Einstein
Mark Twain
Daniel Webster
Anna Pavlova
Sidney Poitier
Richard Simmons
Stevie Wonder

Chapter 10

DEATH AND DYING

For some people, death is not easily discussed. Their feelings about death are too personal, too private to share, except perhaps with their families or close friends. For others, death is a universal link in the cycle of life. It is as much a part of living as birth and it is best acknowledged. Either type of person will find death difficult to face and accept when it strikes someone they know and love.

American culture has to a great extent succeeded in separating life from death. Death is not seen as the natural end of human life, but as an event to be avoided. The subtle societal pressures of this philosophy are an added burden to a person confronted by the death of a loved one. The survivor may feel resentment and anger toward the person who has died.

EVEN BEFORE BIRTH

Most couples realize at some point during a pregnancy that difficulties could occur that would lead to the death of their unborn child. Usually, these difficulties are considered remote possibilities. For the majority of parents-to-be, these fears are transient ones.

For some, however, stillbirth or miscarriage looms as a real threat long before delivery. The effects of toxemia, for example, are cause for concern:

> All your life you hear how important the mother's health is to the baby's normal development. In my case, it seemed by body was working totally against the baby. For most of the seven months I carried Sara, I threw up almost everything I ate. For weeks, I ate nothing. How does a baby survive that?
>
> Then, there was [my prescribed] medication. I took handfuls of pills several times a day. If this didn't kill the baby, what was it doing to her?
>
> Although no one ever said it to me, I knew my baby was given little chance to survive . . . . Death was never mentioned, yet it was always present.

The death of an unborn infant is tragic, especially if the child had been planned for or if the pregnancy follows other difficult birth experiences. A mother who had a miscarriage, a stillbirth and a healthy child before her fourth pregnancy ended at eighteen weeks gestation described her feelings:

> I was very ill for a while and didn't really react to everything until I got home . . . . We became . . . depressed, as the majority of the doctors on my case agreed that we should not have any more children.
>
> We felt abandoned by our friends . . . no one called or visited . . . . Most likely, people were afraid . . . they didn't know what to say or didn't know if we wanted to talk about the experience. It was very difficult for me not to feel resentful and somewhat jealous of friends and strangers who were pregnant at the time.

TOO CLOSE FOR COMFORT

The experiences that parents of premature infants have in the NICU frequently constitute their first encounter with death. The reality there is harsh and violates society's expectations. The lives of many infants are in serious danger but children are not supposed to die.

While a few parents must cope with the possibility of their baby's death before delivery, most have no warning. These parents are suddenly faced with the birth—and possible death—of an infant who may have medical complications the parents never realized could exist, let alone understand.

Yet this tiny human being is tied to them in a special way; it has, after all, already affected their lives for months. The mere thought that this connection, this special relationship, can be so quickly severed often results in fear that can be almost as paralyzing as an actual loss.

This fear is not often expressed aloud, but recognizing their vulnerability during this critical period of their infant's life, some parents are reluctant to become overly involved in its care. They feel that minimal contact will protect them from grief if the child dies. Experts disagree with this thought. Parents, they say, are usually better able to handle the loss if they have tried to know the infant. The procession of thoughts Ryan's mother experienced is common:

> Many times I wondered if Ryan would, could make it. I feared losing him. I would walk away from the hospital wondering if I had to lose him, wouldn't it be easier to lose him now before I became even more attached to him. However, I could never agree to that either. I was already attached beyond belief, and I couldn't stand the thought of losing him.

Parents of premies are often reminded that death is a possibility.

> Just outside the infant care unit, where we "scrubbed up" to go into the nursery, was a sink. Above it was a sheet of paper with a heading that read For Bereaved

Parents. Smaller, lighter print went on to describe the organization, its services, phone numbers, etc. It is difficult for me to admit that I could just never bring myself to really read that page.

"This is crazy," I thought. "Here I am, a rational, mature adult. And I can't even bring myself to read a few words on a sheet of paper—just because it has to do with death." And death was so close. Every day, too close.

When their babies continue to survive, parents often set up their own secret milestones. When the baby attains these goals, immediate fears may be alleviated, but the possibility of death is rarely dismissed during the first months of life.

From the moment he was born, we had to face the possibility of his death. There was no forgetting its threat. Death's name changed with each new problem. Yet death and funerals seemed incongruous with the pastel baby clothes and chiming, smiling toys that filled his nursery at home.

Death was always the shadow cast by every hope. I prayed fervently for his life, but that shadow drove me to plead for time. I begged for time to just see his eyes opened. I wanted time to be alone with him and time to prepare myself for the loss. Even then, I knew there was no way to prepare.

It is not uncommon for parents of infants in an NICU to learn about the death in the nursery of another child whose parents they are acquainted with. This reawakens their own fears that may have subsided.

For parents of twins who have lost one baby, the fear of losing the other baby is unrelenting.

The hardest thing for me was watching other babies grow and get well leaving Robin still in the nursery. It seemed there were a lot of twins who both survived . . . and I felt really cheated to only have had Robin left. It was very hard to spend so much time in the place one baby died wondering if our other tiny daughter would ever really go home.

THE DEATH OF A BABY

Parents whose babies die grieve in their own ways. Most go through similar stages, but in the emotion-filled hours and days immediately prior to and after the death of their infant, they may act in ways unexpected by others.

One mother, who had seven disappointing pregnancies before the death of one of her premature twins, said she had been forced to remain detached from the babies she carried unsuccessfully. One comment made after the death of her baby marked a turning point for this mother:

> When a hospital dietician I [knew] came in and said she was sorry to hear I had lost a son, the walls fell in. In all our struggles to have a family, I had never had a living child die.
>
> I'm sure she doesn't know what a favor she did for me —the only person who acknowledged death. I was shattered . . . depression, catharsis, guilt, you name it.
>
> The nurses stayed away and thoughtfully let my husband stay all hours. What that poor man absorbed, dealing with his own feelings of loss and mine at the same time.

If grieving parents feel the need for special assistance from the hospital staff, they should not hesitate to request it. A mother who had not been allowed to see her dead baby finally insisted upon doing so a day later. The attending nurse recalled what occurred:

> I was called to the mother's room, as she requested to see her baby. I explained to her that the baby was in the mortuary, and at this time the baby would probably have a lot of bruising and discoloration of the skin. She was insistent, even though her husband continued to discourage her. My natural instincts as a mother made me agree with her.
>
> I discussed the situation with her doctor and another supervisor. They could not think of a specific reason why she should not see her baby. I went to the mortuary, dressed and wrapped this cold, heavily discolored baby

and carried her to the mother's room.

I handed the baby to the mother who was sitting in a chair. She was composed and she gently rocked her baby and touched the baby's hands and face. The mother called the baby by her name.

During this time as the mother talked, I listened to her. She explained that when her little boy died from leukemia, she did not see him at the time of death and had always regretted and resented it. This was to be her final pregnancy and she wanted to say a final good-bye to her baby. She said she was now ready to let her go.

I took the baby back to the mortuary, and in my own heart I felt that in the future, I would handle the death of a baby differently. I was able to see the mother accept the grieving process and realized that I had learned a lot from this experience.

Despite separate reactions by two partners, mothers and fathers are usually grateful to learn about an infant's death together. The silent support of knowing that someone else is enduring the same crisis seems to lessen the despair.

When Daryel and I went back to the maternity floor, we told the nurse on duty that our son had died, and I asked if my husband and I could have a cup of coffee in the waiting room because I didn't want to be alone in my room.

We just talked—about the girl's chances, deciding on her name, not giving the boy the name we'd chosen just the evening before because it had never been associated with him. By the time Daryel left to get cleaned up for work, I felt no less shock, but I knew that I could at least face the next few hours without him.

For some parents, their presence at the death of the child provides them with peace of mind concerning the reasons for the child's death. The realization that all efforts were made to save the life of the infant can aid parents working through their grief.

The most important thing to us was that my husband was allowed to be present during the birth of our triplets. The

doctor didn't give us a 50–50 chance that they would
survive at such an early date. The second baby born was
snow white, and we knew immediately that she wasn't
alive.

However, we were able to watch a team of doctors
work on her in the delivery room during the birth of
our third baby who was alive. We know that every
effort was made to bring her around without success. If
I had been asleep or my husband had not been present,
we would have always wondered exactly what had happened.

The question of a "right to die" has stirred numerous contro-
versies in recent years. One mother related an account of a couple's desire that their premature infant be allowed to die peace-
fully:

One of the mothers in our support group had a premature baby with severe problems. After seven months'
hospitalization and numerous surgeries for the infant,
who was still on a respirator, the parents asked the doctor
to allow their baby to die in peace.

The doctor wanted to wait for a few days more, but in
that time the baby experienced irreversible kidney failure so he agreed that they had done all that was humanly
possible for the baby.

He added that he would write orders to remove equipment and not resuscitate, but he had to find a nurse
willing to follow those orders. A day or so later, this was
done and the baby died within a few hours.

The moral and legal considerations for both the parents and the
medical staff in such a decision are tremendous. In some instances, the doctors are legally bound to continue to support life
if prior action to do so has been successful. In other cases, the
policies of a hospital govern both initial and subsequent actions
about life support. In addition, the emotional toll of a parent's
decision to forego further treatment is substantial.

When an infant has been very ill for many months with no
improvement, parents may feel that they could easily accept the

death of their child. They often find that emotional preparation does not lessen the grief.

> On April 18, . . . I came to visit Benjamin as usual. This morning, however, the nurses would not let me in the ICU. Our pediatrician and the chief neonatologist came out to tell me that Benjamin was dying . . . . As much as I had prepared myself for this very event I broke down and cried uncontrollably.
>
> Jim had called the hospital for his daily report and had also received the news. Within minutes, he was with me and we tried to console each other.
>
> The nurses wrapped Benjamin in a blanket and brought him to us. We held him as he rested in absolute peace and for the first time since his birth he was free of the wires and machines.
>
> We both wept. The first feelings were not of grief but rather we were swept by a sense of relief. Were we glad that Benjamin was dead? No, it hurt that he died but we felt glad that he would suffer no more. All the emotional stress of the past five months vanished and we were free to express our grief at having lost our firstborn.

The initial expressions of sorrow and relief demonstrated by this couple were followed by some unexpected emotional outbursts.

> Interestingly, a few weeks after Benjamin's death the pain and frustration Jim and I had suppressed during the preceding five months came to the surface in a flood of emotion. The pain we felt seeing Benjamin suffer, at not having him home with us, the harshness of the hospital, the frustration of not being able to make everything all right suddenly boiled to the surface.
>
> For several days, Jim and I cried a lot or became angry and resentful. However, we soon purged ourselves of these emotional outbursts and were able to see the events of the past months from a new perspective.

It is important for couples to recognize signs of anger, frustration and despondency as part of their grieving. Grief entails much more than tears and sadness.

Death

Oh, death,
how cruel you are.
Hand in hand with fate
you snatched my tiny son.
Noah Asher was his name
We gave him that and so
much of our love
     our hope
     our prayers.
Noah: knowledge of the eternal
Asher: hope and faith.
But names weren't enough.
     Our prayers and our love
     didn't stop your theft.
                              Cindy Hood

Printed by permission of the author

A NOTE TO OTHERS

Perhaps the best advice for those dealing with parents of an infant who has died is this: Do not expect the parents to mourn for their child in a certain way. Some parents direct emotional outbursts toward the medical staff. Others withdraw quietly. It may be difficult for observers to understand the many complexities of a parent's reaction, especially if the observers have never been through a similar experience. Whatever reactions are observed, they are all a result of the parents' efforts to come to terms with their infant's death.

FUNERALS

Arranging for an infant's funeral can be particularly painful. The fact that burial arrangements must be made so soon after death causes added stress. With little time to react emotionally, parents are asked to sign releases so that the child's body can be delivered to a funeral home or so that the hospital can arrange for burial or cremation. An autopsy may be necessary or advisable to determine the exact cause of death. It is difficult to cope with these necessities while still sorting through initial reactions.

> Daryel had a far more black-and-white view of our son's death than I did. The soul was gone; therefore, the body was no longer the person. He had despaired at the intendedly kind suggestion of the funeral director that the funeral parlor dress the body in small baby clothes. "After an autopsy?" he asked, "Don't you get the remains in a plastic bag?"
>
> The closest he came to crying was when he was trying to make the funeral arrangements with our pastor for whom we worked. "I've never had to arrange a funeral before," he said, and then he stood quietly to compose himself before he could say any more words. He said later he felt awkward, not knowing how he was expected to react.

Some parents, on the other hand, find comfort in planning the final arrangements for their child. One mother told of arranging for her daughter's burial:

> I knew funeral arrangements had to be made, and my parents, trying to be helpful, wanted to take over for me. I had to get myself together and realize that if I didn't do things, they would go by without my knowing about them and I would have more regrets.
>
> We wanted everything to be personal because no one had known Windy but us. We had a family plot two hundred miles away where we wanted her to be buried.
>
> The funeral home realized I had had twins and that the other twin was critically ill. They suggested we wait possibly a week just to see how the other baby would do. Two things they pointed out to us: We probably did not want to get that far away from home right now; and if she

were to die, they could bury both of the babies together. This may seem harsh to some people, but not to us. They were just trying to save us the expense and the heartache of going through two funerals.

My family asked me not to view my baby as they felt they would be sparing me, but I was not going to listen. I had to touch her and tell her I loved her once again. This was important to me.

The funeral home also suggested that they could give us a permit to carry Windy to the cemetery with us. Yes, I liked that idea. It was like we were a family—Milton and me in the front seat and Windy in the back seat. There was a peace in the car that is very hard to explain. We had a small graveside ceremony, the funeral was inexpensive and we got what we wanted with no regrets.

ACCEPTING AND ADJUSTING

A death has both immediate and long-range repercussions. The parents who seem resigned and adjusted may find unexpected moments can bring back much pain. Reactions can be triggered by inconsequential events.

When I was feeling low, it seemed like it never failed that I would see twins on TV or in the stores. It was really hard to take. Twins stuck out like a sore thumb. It hurt!

Dreams are an inescapable reminder of the loss of a child. While parents may seem to outsiders to have overcome their grief, they may continue to suffer nightly private terrors.

I would have dreams of both of them being alive, and I was doing motherly chores for them. They were good dreams, but then I would wake up and know that that's what they were, just dreams. The first year was the hardest.

And I thought I was so perfectly resigned. The nightmares started six months after our son's birth. I kept dreaming of boys—strapped to my back, or lying in cribs or needing to be fed. Something must not have been so resigned for me to have those nightmares.

A new offspring can evoke emotions long buried.

Jonathan Christopher, our new son, got the name originally intended for our premature son who died. He's a big, healthy, happy baby. He's probably very different from anything our first son would have been. But he's a boy. Occasionally I look at him and think, "I lost a boy," and feel again that ghost of sadness I've reburied so many times.

MESSAGES OF HOPE

"What can I say to a parent whose baby has just died?" "What can I do for a parent whose child may be dying?" These questions are asked constantly by nurses, doctors, relatives and friends. There are no sure answers. Generally, parents who are adjusting to the loss of their baby do not want others to act as though the infant never existed. They do not want others to assume that a surviving twin can possibly take the place of the twin who died. They do not want to be pushed into creating a "replacement" baby. What parents want—and need—most is understanding and the right to grieve in their own ways without reproach.

Parents usually discover their own answers to problems of adjusting. In this process, they may be helped by a kindly thought or deed or by a sensitive listener. A mother whose son almost died shared a friend's religious message received at a time when the child's survival was uncertain:

"I've been where you are and I know how tough waiting can be . . . but the Lord is holding your hands."

That message came in a card from a coworker as we waited for the doctor's call. We were waiting for everything. Was our four-day-old son alive or dead? Either answer would change our lives forever.

Her understanding of what we "waited" for was genuine. She gave me the hope to believe that our son could live; that God was waiting with us, "holding our hands." Her poignant message was perfect. I am eternally grateful to her.

Death brings difficult lessons to be learned, one of which is that living must go on after an infant's death.

For those next few hours, my husband's experiences and my own were separate. I sat in my hospital room and watched the TV station identification pattern come on. I was numb, almost unthinking.

The first program was providential for me, one of those fifteen-minute meditation programs that tries to touch on reality in one easy lesson. The woman on the program said that our lives are kaleidoscopes, with each day turning up a different pattern. No matter what our experiences are, we get a new chance tomorrow because the pieces fall differently. Each of us remains essentially the same—like the bright pieces of plastic inside the kaleidoscope. But hope can be found in the fact that whether each pattern is more or less beautiful, it is to be experienced only once—and then the pieces move and we go on.

As I was watching the program, Daryel was driving home as the sun was rising. His mind, too, was vacillating between a numb vacuum and random thoughts when one word hit him: dawn. "That would be a wonderful name," he thought. "Dawn. Monica Dawn."

We named our surviving twin Monica Dawn.

Premature

The monitors have stopped.
The deep, triangular concave heaving
of the small chest
simply to breathe
has ended.
Baby Boy B, the second twin,
head badly bruised by forceps
that forced an unwilling victim into air
has dared to desert us,
dared to leave.

I sit here gently rocking a dead child,
whispering half-embarrassed to a body
no longer tied down to life
by the umbilicus of a cold machine,
"It's O.K. . . . It's O.K. . . . "
I, an unlikely first-time mother,
half-breaking numb and only partly grieving
for a boy the doctors raced so desperately
from my womb to tubes
to save.

This we have salvaged:
the pose of a peaceful child,
free of us.

                                        Sherri Nance

AUTOPSY

When a premature infant dies, parents may be asked to give permission to perform an autopsy or, under certain circumstances, an autopsy may be required by state law. In either case, the infant's dazed and saddened parents may be disturbed by the idea of an autopsy or unsure about the decision they make.

Because consent for an autopsy is usually requested immediately after an infant's death, parents may feel pressure to make a decision quickly. They may make a choice they later regret. Parents should be given an opportunity, even if only a brief one, to make their decision in an atmosphere of relative calm.

In Greek, autopsy means "to see with one's own eyes." That is the purpose of the procedure: to attempt to pinpoint the medical cause of death by examining the body carefully where it previously could not be seen.

The procedure is performed by a trained doctor, usually a specialist in pathology, with the same care taken during surgery on living persons. Ordinarily, it is performed at a hospital or similar facility, and a written report is made by the examiner. In some cases, only a partial examination is necessary, particularly if a strongly suspected cause of death can be readily confirmed.

Unless the examination is required by law, an autopsy report is not a public record. Otherwise, it is similar in nature to hospital records and is maintained by the hospital or whatever facility performs the examination. State laws on the availability of reports vary, but a general rule is that parents can obtain a copy, either through their infant's doctor or upon request to the hospital.

However, an autopsy report is not like a death certificate, which notes only the suspected cause of death. It includes much more detail, and it can be upsetting to grieving parents. Because the report's answers or conclusions are generally more important to parents than such detail, it may be wise to ask a doctor to interpret the report.

In trying to make a decision about permitting an autopsy, parents often have conflicting thoughts and feelings. Among these are religious beliefs; the possibility of learning specific information that may relate to any future pregnancies; the possible contribution that may be made to medical knowledge in general or to other parents and their premature infants; and the desire to know for certain why their baby died.

Whatever occurs, parents should be informed about whether or not the law in their state permits a choice about autopsy. If an autopsy is a matter of consent, they should be allowed time to decide and should not be pressured to permit an autopsy if they do not wish it. Whatever parents choose to do should be a decision respected by all concerned.

MAKING FUNERAL ARRANGEMENTS

Because it is often difficult to make decisions at this time, the following suggestions and questions concerning funeral planning were compiled in the hope that they will be of some help to bereaved parents.

When selecting a funeral home, consider its convenience and reputation. It is usually best to select a funeral home that is close to your home. It is also wise to choose one that has been in business for some time and has a good reputation. Ask friends, relatives, a minister, the baby's doctors or nurses for suggestions.

Next, call the funeral homes suggested and ask specific questions concerning their services. If cost will be a factor in your decision, say so. Most funeral directors are willing to work out financial details; if one is not, go elsewhere. After you choose, contact the funeral director and make an appointment to discuss arrangements. Some funeral homes also offer free literature on funeral planning.

Although fathers most frequently make such arrangements, a relative or friend may be asked to assist. Make sure that the person given this responsibility knows exactly what you want and has available all information needed for the death certificate— the parents' full names, social security numbers, home address, place of employment and so forth.

In planning a funeral, consider the following questions:

1. Do you have a cemetery plot? If not, the funeral director can advise you about most local cemeteries. You may wish to choose one near your home because of the mother's health or to make visiting later more convenient. If you have a cemetery plot out of town, it is sometimes possible to arrange for transporting the baby's casket in your own car; a special burial permit may be required in this case.
2. Is burial or cremation preferred?

3. If cremation is preferred, will there be a funeral service beforehand? If so, a casket may have to be purchased or rented, increasing the funeral costs.

4. If burial is preferred, what kind of casket is desired? Caskets can be simple and inexpensive or more elaborate and costly. In some states, there are special requirements concerning burial, such as the mandatory use of a concrete liner or box with a casket. Ask the funeral director about these.

5. Where will the funeral service be held—at a church, the funeral home or at the graveside? Who will conduct the service?

6. Will the casket be closed or open during the service?

7. Will the service be private, with only close family members present, or open also to friends and relatives?

8. What will your baby wear? Do you wish to place sentimental items such as a music box or toy in the casket?

9. Do you wish the death to be announced in your local newspaper? Would you prefer that others contribute to a charitable cause rather than send flowers?

10. Are there any special wishes or needs? For example, if you have not had the opportunity to hold your infant, you may request to do so. The funeral director may be able to provide a room where you can say good-bye to your baby privately. Photographs may also be taken if you desire.

Just reading these questions may be painful, but answers are necessary when a baby dies and parents choose to assume responsibility for planning their infant's funeral. It may be comforting to know that many bereaved parents find that their participation in making final arrangements for their baby is a major step in the grieving process.

Chapter 11

PROFESSIONALS, RELATIVES, FRIENDS, OTHERS

Those who surround parents when birth comes too early—medical professionals, friends, relatives and acquaintances—have a powerful influence on the way parents confront the crisis and cope with it. Parents sense how others expect them to react and these perceptions often affect how well they will handle the stress of having a sick infant in the hospital.

Parents are, of course, not alone with their feelings in this situation. The urgency of the crisis is felt by all involved; the premature birth of just one baby touches many lives.

Doctors and nurses have their own feelings about particular infants, and their parents. Medical professionals are, after all, human. They feel joy and fear, pride and disappointment. Often, parents find them to be understanding and gentle. At other times, doctors and nurses may be so tired and emotionally drained themselves that they can offer little support or encouragement to parents.

Relatives and friends often also have an emotional stake in the birth. Grandparents may ache with helplessness, watching a first grandchild struggle for breath. Friends may be confused by parents' attitudes or fearful of saying the wrong thing. All may feel, along with the parents, the strain of a prolonged hospitalization.

PROFESSIONALS

From their first contact with each other, parents and professionals begin to build a relationship. These first impressions, whether good or bad, become a basis for future communication and dealings. Establishing good rapport is particularly difficult when the situation is so full of stress, but many professionals and parents do develop great respect and trust for one another.

While doctors and nurses must of necessity take the lead in educating parents about their child's medical condition and possible complications of prematurity, those who also exhibit genuine concern for the parents and their emotional health seem to be more effective in communicating with parents and supporting them through the difficult times.

> A premature infant girl, weighing 2 pounds and 3 ounces, was born by Cesarean section at our hospital. The infant had hyaline membrane disease and was placed on a respirator to assist her breathing. As soon as the mother's condition was stable, . . . I wheeled the apprehensive mother into the intensive care nursery . . . . When she saw her tiny infant hooked up to different tubes and machines, she was so overwhelmed she cried.
>
> I explained [about] the equipment that was helping her infant to breathe and suggested that she touch her daughter's hand. She reached out and held the tiny fragile hand. The infant responded by opening her eyes. The mother smiled and whispered, "I think she knows I am her mom." I felt this initial response of mother and

daughter making eye contact was . . . positive . . . [and]
the bonding process had been initiated.

When such sensitive experiences produce positive results, they
give the staff opportunities to reflect on hospital policies and their
own methods of fulfilling their roles. As a result of their experiences with parents, doctors and nurses may decide that changes
are needed. But the sensitive awareness required to evaluate and
react to experiences can be taxing, and demands that professionals must constantly be in touch with their own feelings.

NICU nurses are, in particular, frequently confronted by questions concerning life and death. Many find their attitudes and
beliefs about various issues are challenged each day by events in
the nursery. As one registered nurse commented:

> Health professionals are in a unique position to influence
> how the family emerges from the crisis . . . . In order to
> care effectively for sick newborns and their families, I
> had to explore my own feelings surrounding life and
> death: hardships, joys, sorrow, hope, pride, success, alien-
> ation, love, inadequacies, trust, disorganization, sensitiv-
> ity, fear.

For some nurses, sensitivity towards parents, concern for their
patients and a clear grasp of their own feelings may actually
make their work more difficult. For example, one nurse, recently
assigned to the nursery, "kept waking up in the middle of the
night hearing alarms."

Because becoming emotionally involved with patients carries
certain risks, medical professionals are taught to focus on the
technical aspects of their work in order to limit their own vulnerability. However, when caring for sick newborns, many doctors, nurses and social workers find themselves more personally
involved than they had intended. A pregnant nurse who became close to the parents of a premie under her care commented, "I felt very inadequate . . . because I could hardly talk
to them without crying. They needed support, not tears!"
When the infant died, this nurse questioned her close involvement with the parents even more. Within a short time, how-

ever, her own child was delivered prematurely. After the nurse had returned to work part-time, the mother came back to the nursery to find her.

> She wanted to thank me for caring and helping and told me what her future plans were. She even asked about my child. I don't know how she could remember one person through all the pain, but I've rarely ever felt more positive about my profession.
>
> We are, as professionals, taught and often reminded not to become too involved. It's very easy to do that as one becomes so totally involved in the second-by-second technical aspects of caring for a critical neonate. Perhaps we do hide behind our monitors, respirators and nurses' notes because we are afraid that someone might see us cry. It's nice to know that in the eyes of parents, emotionalism is not a sign of nonprofessionalism. I wonder now if one can ever become "too involved" when working with prematures.

It is difficult, if not impossible, not only for nurses but for all those who deal with parents of premies to keep their personal feelings totally separated from their professional lives. A perinatal social worker spoke of the unique pressures of her role:

> [It is a] struggle, . . . being caught between physicians who can't understand parents' aggressiveness, their reactions of anger, hostility and fear and families who are confused and afraid of medical labels they can't understand, frantically searching for more information, explanations . . . a way to cope with something too overwhelming to comprehend.

A young neonatologist, more familiar with the good outcomes of neonatal treatment during recent years, offered another interesting observation based on his personal vantage point:

> I find it difficult not to be optimistic or hopeful and must control my emotions. If a baby were to die after I had been optimistic, I would be affected by the death, as well

as feeling that I might have made the parents inappropri-
ately hopeful.

When doctors, nurses and social workers succeed in integrating their personal and professional concerns, they often are able
to communicate a sense of human caring to the parents. The
mother of a son born five weeks early with RDS remembered
how good the medical staff made her feel.

> The nurses [gave] me constant progress reports. They
> told me when he was off oxygen and . . . came in to let
> me know he was doing fine. His doctor was at the hospital
> before my husband was down from the delivery room
> and twice more that same night. I found if I asked ques-
> tions, I got answers and I was not made to feel stupid. It
> was important for me to know that people cared and I
> was not just a statistic to them.

Some professionals firmly believe that parents can best handle
the situation if prepared for the worst. As a doctor once told a
parent support group, "At least, you prepare the [parents] for the
worst. And if things are better, you're not going to have any
complaints."

Occasionally, this apparent negativism gives parents the im-
pression that there is no hope for their baby or that the professionals have no concept of what the parents are going through.

> Before she was six weeks old and weighing only 1 pound
> and 5 ounces, we were confronted by [a] doctor [who
> wanted] to take our Catherine off all life-support systems
> to let her "pass" (as the doctors say). We were told then
> that if she did live she would be "a vegetable." With
> mixed feelings and very heavy hearts, we consented and
> waited, and waited and waited . . . she did not "pass."
>
> They sent us to a development specialist to assure us
> we had made the right decision, and we were guaranteed
> the fact that if Catherine did live, she would "never suck
> or swallow, walk, talk and she would be severely cerebral
> palsied." Again we waited.

After two weeks, she began to take milk from a bottle. The doctors were pleased at this, but never [gave] us any word of encouragement. Daily visits to see our angel were never happy for my husband and myself as we knew that each greeting with the doctor meant no word of encouragement for us or Catherine.

We were not told this by just one doctor but all the doctors (from the staff doctor to the specialist outside the hospital). Never a kind word or a reassuring thought that just "maybe" she would live and not be a vegetable. We were told to "put her in a home or at least put her name down for a private home. There's a long list, you know." "You [really] don't want your baby to live." These comments were heard over and over during her 3½ month stay.

There are two sides to a story such as this one. Would the mother have felt the same if her daughter had died? This type of situation—where there are no guarantees—is difficult for both the staff and the parents, no matter what the outcome.

It is also distressing for both the staff and the parents when there are great differences of opinion between them. The reactions of professionals may be interpreted by the parents as disapproval of them and their beliefs.

One day as I reassured the resident . . . that we wanted everything possible done for Victor, he asked if that meant putting him back on the respirator. "No, not that," I responded, "but everything else available." I [added], "I know there are people who think we should just let Victor die."

The doctor replied, "If it were my child, I assure you that's exactly what I would do. But then, he's your baby. If you're willing to assume the costs of an institution, it's your business."

"Have you seen many babies with Victor's problems?" I asked.

"Yes, but they either died or had to be institutionalized," he said.

"Well, I keep praying for Victor," I told him.

He shrugged, [saying] "If that makes you feel better."

Parents who believe that professionals are belittling their attempts to deal with the situation may become withdrawn or angry.

Parent hostility can be especially trying on conscientious staff members who feel the pressures of larger nurseries and increased demands on their time. A neonatologist explained his view.

> Realistically, sick babies come first, and communication must take a lower time priority. The projections of guilt from these parents in a situation "beyond their control" is often expressed as anger towards themselves or the staff. Venting is normal.
>
> We must acknowledge [such] feelings, [but] it is especially frustrating and stressful for physicians and nurses working with long-term sick babies.

In feeling the injustice that their infant is sick, parents may seek out someone to be blamed.

> Parents . . . sometimes concentrate on one thing. I once watched the parents of a premature infant introduce an older sibling to a nurse with, "Here's the nurse who has been sticking your baby."

How do the professionals deal with such hostility? If they are tired and their own emotions are on the surface, they may take such comments as personal assaults. If they can mentally step back from the situation and realize that such words do not come from rational observations but from parental fear, they can attempt to react with understanding.

All professionals who work in the neonatal field may at some point be overwhelmed by the intense nature of their jobs. They must cope daily with the stresses of caring for sick, often critically ill and dying, infants and answering endless questions from worried parents. For them, there is always another baby to care for, always another family that needs attention and answers. A perinatal social worker shared these thoughts with a colleague:

With professionals, the intensity levels are very high, depending on the levels of responsibilities.

Social workers must be where the feelings are. They cannot NOT be moved. They sometimes can't help being overwhelmed.

Each person must find his or her own coping level for keeping the grief inside. In my own case, I let out the sadness and anger I carry inside at other times so that I can function; for example, I might react more intensely to death in a movie. The longer you [are in] practice, the harder it seems to handle those feelings until you get to know the family personally.

I think it's also important to share happiness with people who've been through hell. And let the parents feel cared for by as many people as possible. Some families will get the best support from other team members.

This professional readily acknowledged the emotional burden that the parents must bear:

Whether the baby has been in the hospital two weeks or ten months, the parents who survive "standing up" deserve five stars. This taxes every ounce of coping power. There is a broad range of acceptable behavior, from going crazy to not crying—anything you can do to survive.

Dr. T. Berry Brazelton, well-known pediatrician and author, echoes these sentiments in his advice to parents:

If you can understand your own grieving, you'll have an easier time . . . . You're not alone. Everyone can have the same feelings of craziness and being out of control and then taking it out on the persons with whom they have contact. These are all normal grieving processes.

He hastens to add, however:

Parents should know that as professionals we should settle our own problems with grieving and dealing with babies who don't do well . . . . It's not the parents' responsibility to deal both with their problems and those of the professionals, too. We're just starting to understand ourselves and what parents are going through. But we're learning.

Professionals are often frustrated when confronted by parents who have what professionals may feel are "casual" attitudes towards a serious matter. As one doctor candidly told a group of parents he knew well:

> It shocks me the way you all say, "Well, she was just premature, and she didn't have any problems." I find that . . . I am stunned, [and] I have to [respond], "Listen, that's bad enough." (Dr. Clark Hinkley/Dr. Joseph A. Garcia-Prats)

Parents who exhibit such attitudes may simply be unaware of the potentially life-threatening consequences of prematurity, or on the other hand, they may realize that they are extremely fortunate if their babies do not suffer any long-term handicaps or problems as a result of their prematurity.

Members of the medical team who have had premature infants themselves have a personal perspective of prematurity. They have insight into parental fears and frustrations that their colleagues do not have. One doctor whose wife had premature twins several years ago while he was in training, and whose surviving twin was cared for in a nursery he worked in each day, decided that he would not touch his daughter as long as his wife and other parents were excluded from the nursery. He explained, "I didn't want any accusations of favoritism. I didn't think it would be fair to other parents who couldn't touch their children."

Today, that nursery is open to parents twenty-four hours a day, and the doctor, now a private pediatrician and a member of the hospital's senior staff, still makes rounds in the hospital's special care nurseries when he has a new patient there. This pediatrician has a personal understanding of how difficult it is to communicate with parents under stress. "I estimate that only about 20 percent of what is said to parents gets through to them," he commented.

"That is why I usually repeat myself several times when talking to parents."

All doctors who care for premies would probably agree that communication with a baby's parents is one of the most difficult aspects of their job. They find themselves placed in the position of deciding how and how much parents should be told about their infant's condition. There is a fine line between telling parents "everything" and giving an opinion, between observations and judgments. A doctor expressed some of the issues doctors face in handling communication with parents:

> Black-and-white answers are frequently not available during the course of premie care. The prognosis for the future must be based on experience and statistics depending on the severity of the neonatal course.
>
> However, some prematures whose neonatal course is relatively unremarkable may eventually show poor development, while another premie with a "stormy" neonatal course may do quite well.
>
> It takes months [of] watching a baby to ascertain how well the baby is doing developmentally. No one can assess developmental potential in the first weeks of a premature's life.

Another doctor recalls:

> The child was severely premature, had respiratory distress syndrome and, on the fourth day of life, developed an intraventricular hemorrhage. The child, in spite of his severe complications, managed to survive and did relatively well in the newborn nursery.
>
> The family was advised of the child's progress and the hopes for recovery. However, shortly before discharge, the private pediatrician sat down with the family and informed them that there was an excellent chance that the child was going to be retarded. This came as a complete surprise to the family and was so upsetting that they immediately asked the Neonatology Service to refer [them], on discharge from the hospital, to a different private pediatrician.
>
> Their concern, obviously, was that potential for perma-

nent damage was obvious at the time of the central nervous system bleed and that the presence of actual damage was not discussed until a long time afterwards when
it was obvious that there were some long-term sequelae.

This points out the need for constant and daily discus-
sions with families of sick neonates. I think parents should
be made aware, in the early stages, of exactly what their
newborn's condition is and exactly what the potential
complications can be. Parents placed in similar situations
who have had adequate counseling during the time that
their neonate is so critically ill are much more able to cope
with any new problems that arise in the future.

REFLECTIONS ON A SHRED OF HOPE

In their best moments, doctors and nurses have a grasp of their
own needs, the needs of parents and the facts about a premature
baby's health that allow them to communicate to mothers and
fathers not only information, but also a sense of emotional stability. Such professionals offer parents a way of seeing and relating
to their child, not simply as a sick baby but as a new family
member who needs love and support during a difficult time. A
doctor who worked many years with newborns and is now a
developmental specialist offered some advice to parents whose
premature infants have gone home.

> There's a difference in "being alert to" and "being upset
> about." How one walks that tightrope I don't know. But
> one has to. In all human relationships one walks that
> tightrope. A constantly upset mother cannot hear, can-
> not observe or communicate well with her child. A
> harassed father doesn't communicate good ideas either.
> In a family that lives in a tense, frantic atmosphere, the
> children automatically alert to it and conform to meet
> their own needs. One doesn't learn when tense. One
> doesn't learn to move effectively when one is frightened
> —none of us do. One has to have enough faith to believe
> that the future will unfold and that we will be ready and
> strong enough to meet it when it gets here. (Dr. Murdina
> M. Desmond, "Parenting the Premature Baby)"

When professionals and parents attempt to understand each other, the results can affect the care of future patients. One neonatal nurse reflected on how experiences with parents have changed the policies and procedures in the hospital where she works:

> The biggest change we have made in the approach to parents has been in regard to the care of the dying infant and his family. We are currently applying hospice concepts to our approach with dying infants and their families. This sensitive approach promotes meaningful contact of the family with their dying infant and offers a more comfortable home like environment to the family.

A key word in this nurse's quote is "family." A perinatal social worker outlined the ideal situation:

> If families have a good understanding of the child's medical plan (diagnosis, treatment, and prognosis) and establish good rapport with the medical staff, they will continue to seek good follow-up care and will play an active role in their child's development. As families are encouraged to bond to their infants through participating in their care, and as the child's normal aspects of behavior and care are stressed (as opposed to his birth defect or prematurity), parents will more easily accept the child and begin to cope with the hospital situation. This will help insure that the child receives high-level posthospital care. (Leslie Kane, M.S.W., A.C.S.W., "Critically Ill Newborns: Should The Health Care Team Include Parents?")

Before good rapport can develop, however, both parents and professionals must become aware that their own experiences and emotions affect their reactions to each other.

RELATIVES, FRIENDS AND OTHERS

Medical professionals have an advantage over the relatives, friends and acquaintances of parents of premies—a factual knowledge of events and experiences that can assist them in projecting the most likely outcome of the child's prematurity. Those who do not have such knowledge or experience may feel many of the same emotional conflicts as the parents ("Will the baby live? Will the baby be retarded?") while at the same time trying their best to support the parents.

As a result, the friends and relatives who would normally give support to parents may feel helpless themselves.

Grandparents are among those who feel this conflict most poignantly. One first-time grandmother wrote to her daughter:

> Within hours after the premature birth of the twins, you were talking to me calmly (by phone) and yet you seemed fully aware that both babies might die or develop a handicap. Perhaps you were overly calm which put a burden on me to be as mature as you were being. So, I asked casual questions as though it were a normal situation. It was obvious you and Daryel were operating on faith and did not need pity but our caring and concern.
>
> The outlook for the babies gave me a very heavy heart. When the boy died, we felt the girl had only a small chance. We couldn't indulge that feeling of being grandparents until we saw Monica about seventy days after her birth when she weighed less than 5 pounds and was still in the hospital. We didn't use her name in the family until then.
>
> We had mixed emotions about going to the hospital. [When we arrived] we could hardly believe how healthy Monica was after all she had endured. The anxieties of over two months subsided while watching Monica through the window at the hospital. At those moments of acknowledged life or death, the whole future changes before us.

Another grandmother expressed a question that is often felt:

> As every mother knows, it's so easy to kiss the hurts away when your children are small, but how do you ease their broken hearts when they are adults?

She discussed in detail some of the problems encountered by her son and his wife, admitting the strain she felt by not knowing how to help:

> We stood and watched our son . . . become a superhuman man as he signed a number of papers consenting to treatment for his gravely ill son. The days and months ahead brought more doubts, [but] my husband and I tried to keep a stiff upper lip for the sake of our son and daughter-in-law. They needed all the encouragement anyone could muster for them.
>
> On May 12, our daughter-in-law went into a severe case of postpartum psychosis . . . . Once again, we watched our son sign another mound of papers. As the days, weeks, and dollars rolled by the doctors could give our son no clear-cut answers on either his wife or his son.
>
> After my daughter-in-law was discharged, I felt as though she needed someone with her during the days that followed, but I really didn't want to quit my job. Her doctor seemed to think she would be fine. We wanted to believe that, but we could tell emotional problems still existed. My mind began going like a thrashing machine: "Should I quit my job? Should I ask my son if he'd be more at ease working if I would stay with his wife during the day? Should I ask our daughter-in-law what she preferred? Should I . . . ?" The "Should I?" phrase was like a broken record going around in my mind.

At the same time that grandparents may experience such inner turmoil, they may also have the normal feelings associated with new grandchildren.

> When we peered through the window of the hospital nursery and saw this tiny, precious boy for the first time, our arms ached to hold him. Tender, loving care is necessary for one so small, and that's something grandparents have oodles of . . . .
>
> The day of homecoming arrived. Sitting in the rocker with his sister by my side and this dear little boy in my arms was terrific, marvelous and wonderful.

Other family members encounter similar dilemmas. One woman's sister, who holds a doctorate in child development, described her feelings towards her sister and brother-in-law:

> I was not concerned at that time about the baby; all my anxiety was focused on a concern for Barbie. More than anything in the world I wanted to take her place, even for an hour or two, to give her a short rest from worry and pain.
>
> I felt that my sister was a million miles away emotionally. She was as thoughtful as ever, and almost composed, given the circumstances. My brother-in-law was carrying on as usual, as if nothing had really changed yet. His way of coping was to keep going on as normally as possible.
>
> Our offerings and givings of help, as in-laws, were so great that at times I am sure we caused my sister and brother-in-law conflict and discomfort. Each member of the [two] families involved had a somewhat different idea of what was best and what the appropriate boundaries between generational families should be. Despite the pressure which these differences may have placed on them, both [my sister and her husband] tolerated the constant involvement of concerned relatives with considerable patience and, at times, welcomed it.

Another young woman expressed the frustration of watching an in-law deal with the agony of realizing that his child's life was endangered:

> Chet, whose gentle, loving spirit never ceases to amaze me, seemed much like a bewildered, weaponless soldier in the midst of fierce battle. I felt so helpless. I wanted to share those agonizing moments with him—in some way lighten his burden. But I knew all too well that he was separated from the entire world at that moment and to enter into his plane of space would have been intrusion.

One of Chet's friends recalled his reaction to the news of Zachary's early birth:

Chet was telephoning us. (How nice. I like to hear from Chet.) Hello, Chet. What's new? Sherry had the baby. Really?! Great! Oh, wait a minute, it's not time yet.

Chet told me the whole story. Long labor. Sherry vomited. Special hospital. Tubes. No holding. (How tight he is. They need help.) I could come to Houston. No, nothing you can do. Thanks for listening. Yes, said Chet, I'll try to sleep (Why do I feel like someone died?)

On the day following Ryan's birth, a friend of his mother called. She sensed the worry in Ryan's mother's voice and reacted:

> I wanted to cry, but I knew that sometimes friends need to be strong, need to be supportive. I spoke the necessary encouraging words to her and asked that she pass these same words of encouragement to Dick.
>
> But I thought to myself, "Will this baby make it?" How could fate, how could God let this happen to two people who I knew would be "perfect parents?" Special prayers were said . . . . I often thought to myself: This baby must live!

A SISTER'S VIEW

Some relatives or friends are able to offer just the right words at just the right times to make the parents feel less alone. Friends, in particular, can impart the emotional equilibrium that only an objective bystander can give.

> Ironically, Sharon and I had talked about when she and Tim would start their childbirth classes the day she went into premature labor, months before they were ready. As soon as the phone rang the next morning and I heard Tim's voice, I knew her pregnancy and the baby were in trouble . . . . It was obvious that this tall, capable lawyer had been reduced to [feeling] lost and totally helpless in the situation. In Tim's voice there was concern and sadness, not the joy of "It's a girl" or "We're here and it's happening and Sharon is fine." There were no cigars or candy, just lots of coffee.
>
> I met Tim later outside Sharon's room, and both of us

felt inadequate. Since we had lots of friends who had had lots of babies under all sorts of situations, [my husband] Joe and I were more familiar with the techniques and terms used now than these first-time parents. We could ask more in-depth questions and remember the answers better later on.

My husband was with Tim the next day when Susan was brought out from delivery and her small size, 2 pounds and 15 ounces—a doll in reality—was brought home. The sigh of relief at her being alive and well was a communal one but short-lived as she developed classic respiratory problems . . . and was transferred to [another hospital].

This friend continued to help by running errands, calling to ask how things were and offering encouragement whenever the parents seemed depressed. She also gave her own form of support to Susan:

As a mother familiar with the run-of-the-mill 6- or 7-pounder, I could see Susan as a "real" baby and as a creature who needed the "personification" that Tim and Sharon were afraid to give her because of the fear of losing her . . . . Blind to the "forest," I saw Susan as a little "tree," a cousin to my kids, entitled to the privilege and rights therein. Those included her first dolly, a scaled-down version of Holly Hobbie, her first Easter basket, and a real Easter sunsuit—PERSONALIZED with her name and daisies and handsewn by me, with a note that she could keep it for her dollies when she was older. It was probably a subconscious effort on my part to project her safely into their family's future, past all this trauma.

Not all friends are so understanding. A childbirth educator who had a premature baby was saddened by the reactions of her friends and relatives:

Some relatives were fearful of getting "close" to the situation, apparently to protect their emotions and feelings. This hurt me. Chelcee was a member of our family . . . . If her mother wasn't fearful of her life, I felt no one else should react to her as a freak of nature barely surviving.

I think this is an interesting point to prepare couples for. Your friends and relatives will react to your situation on both ends of the spectrum. The extremes will be universal support and encouragement or total awesome indifference. People on the whole do not know how to honestly react to an abnormal situation with any degree of normalcy.

Perhaps those who are most able to relate to parents of premature infants are other parents of premies. They can listen past the talk of monitors and wires to hear what the real problems of the infants are, see past the oxygen hoods and N/G tubes to view the normal aspects of the babies. No one can ever give the same support as that offered by a person who has survived a similar situation. A new grandmother wrote her daughter:

> Our fear and panic take over when we focus in on our own limitations. This is why the premie group serves such a good purpose. The burden is shared; others assist in carrying you beyond your own limits.

But other parents of premies are also human. They have not always experienced exactly the same events as those they endeavor to support and they may not always know the best manner of listening. A member of a parent support group expressed her concerns regarding one of her contacts:

> I answered the phone. A woman's voice said, "I just had a premie. Do you ever get over this depression?"
>
> We talked quite a while. She expressed a reluctance to visit her baby. I sensed an underlying feeling that she intuitively knew her baby would not survive, although she was quite cheerful about his progress. But I encouraged her to have hope and to get to know her baby. There are no guarantees in life whether the baby is sick or healthy. We can only live a day at a time and make the best of each moment.
>
> She began visiting the baby. I called her, took her

literature and clothing. I notified the social worker at the hospital where her baby had been transferred. Two weeks later, I heard that the baby had died. Unable to reach her by phone, I sent a card and note. We've not been in touch since.

I think about her often. Did I do the right thing? Was it wrong to give her hope? Should I have done more? Or was it best that she did try to get to know her baby even though, realistically, his chances were poor. I don't know the answers. Maybe the answers are different for each of us.

PERSPECTIVES

Just as a normal, full-term birth brings together many people, so too does an unexpected birth. But the lives of parents, medical professionals, relatives and friends are touched in a different way when the birth is premature and the infant requires special care. The experience highlights for each individual his or her own vulnerabilities, and it calls for all those affected by the birth to find within themselves the courage to face this crisis.

For concerned parents, the kind words and cautiously optimistic comments of others are keys to their emotional survival.

> I think of my husband, who has listened to me cry. I think of Lee, who as godmother bounced my kid on her knees and helped her be "normal." I think of Margaret, who listened, and helped me to arrive on time for the strict visiting periods. I think of the doctor who punctured and ruined a sterile pack of tubing while drawing diagrams of the renal system so that I could have a grasp of what acidosis really was. I think of the doctor who is the head of two departments in a major medical school who dropped by the premature nursery before leaving for home because his wife told him that I really wanted answers to some questions about my baby. I remember the cleaning lady in the hospital who talked to me of birth and death as she mopped the floor the morning my son died. I think of the nurses who told me confidential

stories that possibly should not have been told, so that I could put my own experience in perspective. I think of Sherry, and Patty, and Ella Beth, and Susan, and Leslie and all the others who first made me feel that there were other people with whom I could share the craziness of a not-exactly-but-almost-normal situation.

They were my tickets to sanity during very difficult times.

Into Your Hands
(A tribute to the newborn intensive care nurse)

Into your hands I bring a life,
Small and fragile
just a spark that's fading
in the dawn and yet as precious as any.

For I have learned from you
that all life is right
and justifies the greatest fight
that man can give to save it.

That it may be wasted later is true;
but to you here and now,
It is tended and nurtured with infinite skill and
*   wisdom,*
until every energy for life which man can give has
*   been expended.*
For you, death is still the archintruder;
common as he is he has not dulled your senses.

For I have seen your tears,
and I have seen you soar when one wee name was
*   stricken from his list*
And I have felt your strength—
those strong, broad shoulders bearing
great burdens gently.
For you have pitted brain and skill and love alone
*   against the night and won.*

I have listened to your instinct
that wild and magic unmeasurable something
that men do not possess.
Pending and mothering and feeling and knowing
*   when something's wrong.*
When all else of man's devices fail to know.

So once more . . . into your hands I bring a life.
Small and fragile; just a spark that's fading in the
*   dawn.*
For who but you can hold this life secure . . .
and who but you can know how great a triumph may
*   yet await*
Another dawn.

Alan Van Orman, M.D.
Pediatric Resident 1968 to 1970
University of Utah
Medical Center
Salt Lake City, Utah

Parent's reactions to the inevitable death of their infant generally fall into three categories. One group of parents clings desperately to hope for survival, though aware of reality. A second
group of parents has an intense desire to discontinue therapy;
they surrender to the inevitable. A third group of parents is
bewildered and totally dependent on professional guidance. Although this categorization oversimplifies the variations, it does in
fact describe the vast majority of parents.

Most parents seem to fall in the first category: They cling desperately to a thread of hope whether or not the physician offers
it. They often feel that giving up hope is tantamount to executing
their baby.

A recent experience with a mother of a thanatophoric dwarf
is instructive. Thanatophoric dwarves live only a few hours, or at
most several months. None have been known to survive. This
infant was maintained on a ventilator for several weeks until his
death. Several house officers and a number of consultants stated
repeatedly to this intelligent mother that her infant would not
survive; in fact, there was no hope. There were indeed accurate
statements. One consultant raised the idea of autopsy while the

infant was still being sustained successfully.

The mother kept a constant vigil. She was sufficiently intelligent to understand the significance of respirator settings and she intensely followed the changes. She repeatedly inquired about improvement and she was repeatedly told that the baby would die. After a week or ten days, with exasperation and considerable emotion, she confronted the social worker. She was tired and angry with the repetitive pronouncements of predicted death. Her capacity to deal with the situation depended on a little hope, whether or not this was justified. She insisted that we maintain maximum effort, regardless of "what the doctors thought" of the outcome. In deference to her needs, we spared no effort. The baby died several weeks after admission to the nursery.

This mother was one of few who actually voiced her exasperation with hopelessness and with repeated pronouncements of inevitable death. Complete honesty can sometimes be brutal. In the circumstances just described, honesty could have been maintained far more gently by preserving the shred of hope this mother needed so desperately. Well aware of the inevitability of her infant's death, she nevertheless cried out for life support. A large number of parents feel identically, but remain silent. They need the last shred of hope, and they need to know that their infant died in spite of a maximum effort to maintain life.

Dr. Sheldon Korones
Chief of Neonatology
University of Tennessee
Health Sciences Center
Memphis, Tennessee

Every part of life is intrinisically and inseparably bonded to that environment which supports it. A fish removed from water is only a limp and impotently pulsating mass of protoplasm; a lion deprived of his jungle in which to stalk his prey is robbed of his identity as head of the animal kingdom, indeed of his very means of existence. He looks displaced and incomplete strutting [about] his barred cage in the zoo. Likewise, the 5½-month fetus is bonded to his mother's womb. There his tiny limbs, wrinkled skin, underdeveloped lungs, still sealed eyes are all the proper part and parcel of his existence. The outside world into which Ryan was wrenched at so early an age, however, has far more exacting demands. Thus, gazing upon him those first few days was difficult. He looked out of place. He was too small, too under-developed. I wanted him to reenter my sister's womb and not come out for another 3½ months. It's what Marcia and Chuck wanted too. If Ryan had been given any choice he probably would have wanted it as well. But none of us were given any choice. The only choice, the only option, was to cope with the situation at hand in whatever way we could. Hence began months of patient, desperate coping.

Chapter 12

WHAT ABOUT THE NEXT TIME?

*The first time you have a premie is heartbreaking, because
whether or not you are surprised or forewarned you are just
so darn ignorant about premature babies and the whole
lifesaving concept.
The second time it's heartbreaking because you learned so
much the first time, enough to know the worst that can
happen.*

These words were written by a mother whose first pregnancy
ended in miscarriage and who subsequently had a premature
son. An unplanned third pregnancy abruptly ended this couple's
worries of deciding whether or not to have another child.

For some parents, the extended anxieties of having an ill or
hospitalized baby are a burden they refuse to shoulder again. On
the other hand, others are willing to assume whatever risk is
involved in having another child.

FACTORS INFLUENCING A DECISION

1. The risk of another premature birth: When the cause of prematurity is unknown, a woman has a 25 percent chance of delivering another baby prematurely. Even when a reason for the prematurity can be given and steps can be taken to lessen the chances of another premature birth, delivery may occur early again.

2. The severity of the problems of the premature infant: A couple who has had a critically ill infant may need time to adjust to the child's needs. Parents may still feel stress, especially if the child has long-lasting problems or handicaps.

3. The death of a child: A couple whose infant dies may be advised to try immediately to have another baby. However, a new joy cannot mask past grief. Grief must be felt, analyzed, understood and integrated by each person who has faced the death of a premature infant.

4. The physical and emotional health of the mother: Even today, women die in childbirth. Those who come close to dying but survive have a different outlook on pregnancy than other women who had a relatively easy pregnancy and delivery.

   Some active women cannot emotionally handle the weeks or months of bed rest that may be necessary with a high-risk pregnancy. A working woman may have reached a point where such a long time away from her work would be detrimental to her career or cause her to lose her job.

5. Marital and family stress: The way each family member dealt with the premature birth, the current work status of spouses, child care arrangements and many other personal matters affect decisions about childbearing. Questions regarding sexual intercourse—including the need for contraception or the possibility of medically required abstinence during a subsequent high-risk pregnancy—are not easily answered.

6. Family size: Each parent has the concept of an ideal

family size tucked away consciously or unconsciously. For some, one child is enough; others want more, but may reconsider their initial plans after having a baby prematurely.

7. Attitudes of friends and relatives: Relatives and friends can exert either subtle influences or heavy pressures about family size or additional pregnancies. The decision, however, is for the couple alone to make. A couple should realistically consider that help from friends and relatives may be necessary during a high-risk pregnancy or if another premature delivery occurs.

8. Financial worries: Parents who anticipate major difficulties with the large bill that can result as hospital costs rise are less likely to attempt another pregnancy. If they decide to try again, they should research the types of insurance that provide coverage for major problems.

9. Professional opinions: Many professionals would advise a woman who has a history of high-risk pregnancies not to become pregnant again. Various examinations and tests can assist the high-risk woman who wants children in making a decision about pregnancy. Second or third professional opinions may also be helpful.

10. Moral, religious or ethical implications: Moral, religious or ethical questions may be raised about contraception, abortion, heroic life-saving procedures or the long-term consequences and costs to society of raising a potentially handicapped child. There are no easy answers to these questions. The power to create life carries with it an awesome responsibility.

THE DECISION TO HAVE NO MORE CHILDREN

Some couples have no choice about having more children because of subsequent infertility, a necessary hysterectomy or a medical condition that precludes pregnancy. For others, the deciding factors are not medical, but personal. No matter what the basis of this decision, couples may be torn between disappointment in ending their childbearing years and relief in having made a final decision.

> My problems started with nausea. I knew I was pregnant before I could take a pregnancy test. In the last part of my fourth month, I developed chest pains . . . . When I went for my six-month checkup my blood pressure was high, I was leaking protein into my urine and I was losing weight. I weighed 123 pounds when I got pregnant; now I weighed 114.
>
> I was given medication for my blood pressure and for headaches. I had a reaction to the medicine. They put me on an IV to try and stop the vomiting.
>
> I had been told that once the baby was delivered, I would be fine. No one told me there is a forty-eight-hour critical period after a toxemia delivery. I developed the complications. My hospital did not have an intensive care unit so they kept me in the labor and delivery [room] for two days.
>
> My nephrologist said most people who have pregnancies like mine abort in the third or fourth month. He also said I had symptoms he had only read about.
>
> We wanted another baby but we had to consider the baby's health and my own health. There was no way to know whether or not I could survive another pregnancy.
>
> Also, it seemed Sara was a gift from God. He had made sure she survived those months inside of me and He gave her the strength to survive the difficult months in the hospital. Would the next baby be so lucky?
>
> Another factor is my age. If we wanted to plan another baby, we would have had to quickly do so. I didn't feel I was physically or emotionally ready to go through another high-risk pregnancy just a year after the first.
>
> A decision had to be made. Having my tubes tied was so final. I would never be able to have another baby.

> After enduring a tiring, traumatic first year with Karen, my husband and I were definite about the fact that two children were all we wanted.
>
> Since our daughter was considered at high risk for the first year of life, we decided to forego any permanent

form of birth control. But when she was eighteen months old, I had a tubal ligation.

One thing we had considered is that we would want no more children if anything happened to ours. We would have to deal with that if it happened and get on with life.

The relief that we have experienced since the surgery is indescribable. The decision for sterilization was not one made in haste, and we in no way regret it.

The continuing advances in perinatology may someday allow parents like Jonah's mother to make different decisions from those they now feel they must make:

Because the reasons for the prematurity are as yet unexplained, thus implying a possible tendency, I feel it would be too risky to subject another baby to such a traumatic beginning.

INDECISION

Susan's mother is like many women who, with their husbands, are delaying the decision about having more children:

Frankly, I don't know if there will be another pregnancy for me or not.

We were fortunate that Susan was a strong baby and overcame the initial problems caused by her prematurity, but the fear that we may not be so lucky the second time around is ever present.

While it is true in many cases that one premature birth does not mean that another will follow, I happen to believe that the odds are against me.

For one thing, I am already thirty-three and I had great difficulty in becoming pregnant the first time. Also, my doctor has confirmed that I am a DES daughter. We must consider all the ramifications of that fact.

Because our respect for human life goes deep, the decision will not be easy.

Such indecision is not uncommon. It often takes some time after a premature birth for parents to feel they are ready and able to make a rational or objective decision about a subsequent pregnancy.

A DECISION: YES

Some couples consciously decide that they do want more children. For others, an unplanned pregnancy may end the need to make a decision. Although a few parents choose to attempt another pregnancy immediately, most postpone their plans for a time.

But Not Now

Although some women become pregnant so soon after having a premature infant that there is no opportunity to weigh alternatives, the majority of parents take measures to prevent having a baby right away. They feel they need a breathing space, a time to catch up with the world and relax with their children. So much of the "premature experience" deals with the necessity of coping with events and caring for the new baby that parents often find it difficult simply to enjoy living during that stressful time. Eventually, all parents discover they need to develop a new self-image, one in which their child's needs and their own are balanced.

Many psychologists favor the spacing even of healthy term infants. For varied reasons, parents of premature or ill infants often consider waiting even longer than may be recommended.

> I've always said that I wanted more children, but I now keep pushing forward the time that I want to be pregnant again. If I had become pregnant during those first years before all the medical bills were paid, I'm not sure how well I would have handled the situation. The scares that I had twice when I was under stress and my menstrual cycles went completely crazy were bad enough.

But I'm realizing more and more that I only now have time to relate to my husband in some of the ways that we planned all along. I became pregnant so soon after our marriage and have had so many responsibilities since, that it has been hard at times to redefine our goals as husband and wife.

I want more time to be creative—to write, do calligraphy and sing. It's hard to be creative when the demands of an infant only allow your private time to be early in the dawning when you may be too tired to care about creativity.

Pregnant Again

Once a definite decision is made to have another baby or once a pregnancy occurs and is not terminated, a couple must make several major decisions. They first need to be secure in their choice of a doctor and a hospital.

The obstetrician should be able to manage a high-risk pregnancy or, if necessary, be able to refer the woman to an obstetrician who specializes in problem pregnancies.

> I decided to remain with the same obstetrician who had seen me through my last pregnancy and premature delivery because I had established some rapport with him. In discussing my new pregnancy, although the cause for prematurity was still uncertain, we decided to take several precautions this time. He approved my SPUN diet, agreed to a McDonald stitch, recommended ultrasound and a maternity corset—and he really listened to me and examined me whenever I felt I had a problem.

Some women are dissatisfied with the explanations and information given them by the obstetrician who delivered their premies. They may find it helpful to get second or third opinions from other doctors.

> My obstetrician virtually told me I had a miscarriage that lived. He said it could happen to anyone. Well, I didn't believe him. After pouring [out] my heart and personal

account [to several other] doctors . . . . I found I had a bicorneal uterus plus an incompetent cervix.

I found out about my malformed uterus through a hysterosalpingogram. The radiologist and obstetrician described this as a test given to women who have had three or four miscarriages or lost babies. How ridiculous! . . . Why have several miscarriages?

[Many] obstetricians have not spent days and weeks over a child's Isolette, hoping the baby will live. [That is] a situation I never want to be in again.

I must have surgery to repair my uterus, a suture to tighten the cervix and a Cesarean delivery next time but at least I know what happened to me and that I have a chance for another baby.

If I had not taken the initiative to follow up on my own . . . situation, no doctor would have. Two . . . told me, "Don't worry, just try again." I now know I would have [given birth to] another extremely premature baby. I'm glad I sought second and third opinions.

Others who decide to change doctors may at first feel hesitant.

I believed that changing doctors in mid-pregnancy was forbidden, but my second pregnancy did not go well. It ended at twenty-seven weeks. Somehow the doctor I had was not quite right for me. I felt that his examinations were not as complete as they should have been. He did not show much interest in my pregnancy.

I considered changing doctors but I was too embarrassed. Would the doctor I left and the new doctor both think I was stupid?

During my third pregnancy, I had the same feelings about my doctor. At three months, I finally decided to change doctors, no matter what anyone thought.

One important lesson I learned is that if you think things aren't going the way they should, you should at least get a second opinion. If you find that the doctor you are going to isn't right, then change. It's your body and your baby.

HIGH-RISK OBSTETRICS

High-risk obstetrics is a commonly used term for the field of medicine known as maternal-fetal medicine or perinatology. It is a specialty offered in most medical schools.

Before a woman is classified as a high risk for pregnancy, a variety of factors, including a history of premature birth, is considered. Doctors do not automatically categorize a woman who has delivered one baby prematurely as a high risk.

A high-risk woman who becomes pregnant should carefully choose both the doctor who will handle her prenatal care and delivery and the hospital where she will deliver:

1. If there is a medical school in your area, call and ask for the names of local doctors specializing in maternal-fetal medicine who are affiliated with the medical school but also have their own practices. Ask if the medical school operates a high-risk obstetrics clinic.
2. If there is a support group for parents of premature infants in the area, call one or more group members and ask for their suggestions.
3. Call or visit hospitals in the vicinity. Ask about their nursery facilities—the levels of nurseries, staffing, number of beds, nurse-to-baby ratio, visitation policies and so forth.
4. Consider the location of the hospital. How far away is it? Would getting to the hospital in traffic be a problem if an emergency arose?
5. Check to see how many of the doctors suggested are affiliated with the hospitals you like best.
6. Call several doctors' offices and inquire about fees, patient load, associates and so forth. When you have made a preliminary choice, call and make an appointment to meet the doctor. Your husband may want to accompany you.
7. During the appointment, be sure to give the doctor your complete medical history and ask specific questions about the doctor's usual practices in handling a high-risk patient.

The choice of a hospital is usually tied to the choice of a doctor, since most physicians are affiliated with one or two local hospitals, but not all. Keep in mind that a hospital associated with a medical school usually offers the most comprehensive facilities for neonatal care. If another premature birth occurs, it is best for delivery to be in a hospital with good neonatal facilities rather than having to rely on transport of the baby to a regional perinatal center or a hospital that has an NICU. Also, if labor begins early, the doctory may advise the pregnant woman to go to a hospital with an NICU.

MANAGEMENT OF A HIGH-RISK PREGNANCY

Candidates for high-risk pregnancies include women who have diabetes, thyroid disease, hypertensive disorders, Rh negativity, persistent bleeding or a history of miscarriages or premature births. It is important for women with these problems to discuss openly with their doctors the manner in which their care will be handled in the event of conception. Women should also ask their doctors about the medical tests and procedures now available, including:

- A hysterosalpingogram, where a radiopaque substance is injected into the uterus and ovaries before conception to diagnose uterine abnormalities that may have contributed to a premature delivery.
- McDonald, Shirodkar, Wurm or Lash sutures, which are surgical stitches intended to keep the cervix closed for the duration of a pregnancy.
- Sonography (known as ultrasound, Beta Scan, sonogram, Sonargram), where high-frequency sound waves are used to produce a picture of the uterus, placenta and fetus. This technique is used to determine gestational age, multiple births or placental abnormalities; some birth defects can also be diagnosed before delivery.
- Amniocentesis, where a needle is inserted through the abdomen and uterus into the amniotic sac and fluid is removed for analysis. Laboratory tests on the fluid can

help doctors assess fetal health and maturity, as well as
aid in diagnosing maternal problems (such as hydramnios) that may result in premature delivery.

Doctors may also advise a couple to seek genetic counseling if
there is evidence of genetic birth defects in addition to
prematurity. Like neonatology and perinatology, the field of genetic counseling is relatively new, and there are many tests and
procedures available now that did not exist a few years ago. As
advances in perinatology and genetic research continue, there
will undoubtedly be even more means of aiding high-risk women
in conceiving and carrying a healthy baby to term.

Even when various tests and procedures are done, there are
worries. One mother scheduled to have a McDonald stitch was
concerned enough about the effects of the anesthesia to be used
that she discussed the matter with the anesthesiologist before
surgery. The doctor reassured her that the baby would not be
harmed, but the mother continued to be concerned about the
surgery itself. She and her obstetrician discussed the various
drugs she would be given following surgery. She was told that
after she awoke from surgery she would be allowed to listen to
the baby's heartbeat:

> I had been told that someone would come with a feto-
> scope to check the baby's heartbeat. No one came. I
> asked several times and was told "soon." By 6 p.m., I
> demanded to know how soon. The nurse called me on
> the intercom to say they had just checked and needed a
> doctor's order to get a fetoscope since they didn't have
> one at the station. They were unable to reach my doctor
> at that time, so I was to remind him the next day.
>
> I had not felt my baby move so I was becoming anxious.
> I decided to call my doctor's telephone answering ser-
> vice and explain the situation. I made the call at 7 p.m.
> and within half an hour, two labor and delivery nurses
> arrived with an amplifying fetoscope. The three of us
> listened intently, and after much maneuvering and
> many sounds, the baby's heartbeat sounded a reassuring
> thump, thump, thump.
>
> The nurses were pleasant and understanding, and I felt

much better for having the reassurance of hearing my baby. That night I slept more easily knowing the life inside me was beating.

DIET AND DRUGS DURING PREGNANCY

Inadequate diet during pregnancy can cause premature birth, low birth weight, stillbirth, infant mortality and various problems for the child. Poor diet is specifically associated with metabolic toxemia of late pregnancy (MTLP), abruptio placentae, anemia, hypertension and frequent maternal infections. Although improper diet does not always cause these problems, evidence indicates that a pregnant woman's diet is of enough concern—especially in a high-risk pregnancy—to warrant careful consultation and planning with her doctor.

A pregnant woman should concentrate on quality calories rather than empty ones. The kind of food she eats is more important than how much she gains. Excessive weight gain is, however, not advisable. A complete, inexpensive, nutritional diet—approved by the American Red Cross and numerous obstetricians —has been formulated by the Society for the Protection of the Unborn Through Nutrition (SPUN). For more information, contact the Society for the Protection of the Unborn Through Nutrition, 17 North Wabash, Suite 603, Chicago, Illinois 60602.

A Sound Diet for Pregnancy (adapted from SPUN publication, *Preventing Nutritional Complications of Pregnancy: A Manual for SPUN Counselors,* 1978, and *How To Be a Healthy Mother and Have a Healthy Baby,* 1980.)

During pregnancy, women need more of good quality foods than when they are not pregnant. To satisfy the nutritional stress of pregnancy and provide for her baby's growth, it is crucial for every mother to have, *every day,* at least:

1. One quart (four glasses) of milk: whole, low fat, skim, or powdered skim milk or buttermilk. Natural

cheese, yogurt or cottage cheese can be used as sub-
stitutes for milk.

2. Two eggs.

3. Two servings of fish, chicken or turkey, lean beef,
veal, lamb, pork, liver or kidney. For each serving of
meat, 4 ounces of cheese or 6 ounces of cottage
cheese can be substituted.

Alternative means of obtaining complete proteins
include the following combinations: (*Diet for a Small
Planet,* by Frances Moore Lappe.)

Brown rice with beans, cheese, seeds or milk.

Corn meal with beans, cheese or milk.

Beans with brown rice, whole grain noodles or
milk.

Peanuts or peanut butter with sunflower seeds or
milk.

Whole wheat bread or noodles with beans, cheese,
peanut butter or milk.

4. Two servings of fresh, green leafy vegetables: mus-
tard, beet, collard, dandelion or turnip greens; spin-
ach, cabbage, broccoli, parsley, kale or Swiss chard.

5. Two choices: a whole potato, large green pepper,
grapefruit, orange, lemon, lime, papaya or tomato.
(One large glass of juice may be substituted for a
piece of fruit.)

6. Five servings of whole-grain breads, rolls or cereals
(such as granola). Other nutritious grain products include wheat germ; oatmeal; buckwheat or whole
wheat pancakes or waffles; corn tortillas; corn bread;
corn, bran, or whole wheat muffins; and brown rice.

7. Three pats of butter or the equivalent in oil.

Also include in your diet:

8. A yellow or orange vegetable or fruit at least five
times a week.

9. Liver once a week.

10. Salt: SALT YOUR FOOD TO TASTE.

11. Water: Drink to satisfy thirst.

12. Vitamin/mineral supplements. Supplementation
should be used only as *insurance,* not as a substitute
for foods.

When mothers follow this diet plan, they will be obtaining every day approximately 2,600 calories, at least 80 to 100 grams of high-quality proteins, and all other essential nutrients in amounts sufficient for pregnancy. It is important to note, however, that no two pregnant women have identical nutritional requirements. Women who are underweight, are experiencing undue stress or were previously undernourished have even more pronounced nutritional needs during pregnancy.

The mother with twins has dramatically increased needs. She requires at least 30 grams more protein and 500 additional calories (which can easily be provided by an extra quart of milk per day or its equivalent in other complete proteins) above the normal pregnancy requirements.

There are a number of foods you should not eat because they do not provide you with the nutrients you need to build your baby. You should avoid white bread and rolls; bleached cornmeal; soda pop; commercial pies, cakes, cookies and doughnuts; candy; other snacks of limited value; ice cream; most commercial cereals and many other packaged foods; beverages and foods that contain caffeine; and hot dogs and luncheon meats (which don't have the value of the meats they replace and which have chemicals that might endanger your baby's health). All of these foods and added sugar (brown or white) have very little nutritional value and can rob you of important nutrients you need. Another reason to avoid them is that they will fill you up with empty calories and take the place of the good foods that you and your baby need.[2]

When pregnant or planning to become pregnant, a woman should avoid any weight-loss diet, diuretics or drugs of any kind. No prescription or over-the-counter-drug has been proved to be 100 percent safe during pregnancy.

TREATMENT OF PREMATURE LABOR

Even with the best precautions, a mother may go into premature labor. New methods of stopping premature labor and prolonging pregnancy have been developed in recent years. In the past, bed rest, sedatives, hormone inhibitors and various drugs, including alcohol, were prescribed in attempts to prevent early labor. However, growing concern over possible side effects to the fetus resulting from the use of alcohol, and the fact that other methods of treatment have been only partially successful prompted researchers to continue to seek better answers.

One result of this research was the discovery that a group of drugs called betamimetics, or smooth-muscle relaxants, is useful in halting labor by relaxing the smooth muscles of the uterus. In 1980, the U.S. Food and Drug Administration approved the use of one betamimetic, ritrodrine hydrocloride (known commercially as Yutopar), specifically for treatment of premature labor. Other types of betamimetics have been used abroad for several years and a few, primarily terbutaline (Brethine), have been used experimentally in the United States.

> When we were transferred to Longview to look for a house, I started having contractions. My husband took me to the emergency room at the hospital and I was admitted since our unborn baby was at twenty-eight weeks gestation.
>
> I was frightened and scared, and both of us had tears in our eyes since the hospital did not have an NICU. I was lucky since the obstetrician started me on intravenous drip of Brethine to prevent premature birth. I was in the hospital for ten days of bed rest and took Brethine orally. After discharge, I was in bed until the baby was at thirty-six weeks gestation. . . . Today I'm still pregnant at thirty-eight weeks gestation.
>
> [*Editor's note:* Shortly after this was written, this mother gave birth to a healthy baby boy, named Joey, who weighed 8 pounds and 8 ounces.]

Sometimes the onset of labor signals that the infant is in distress or that the mother's life is endangered. Stopping labor in these cases may prove more harmful than premature birth, especially if the infant will have immediate access to the facilities of an

NICU. In most cases, however, doctors do take steps to halt labor and to prolong the pregnancy.

Because a major concern when premature labor occurs is the maturity of the infant's lungs, which are among the last organs to develop, a doctor may order a test done to determine lung maturity. Amniotic fluid is removed by amniocentesis, and the fluid is analyzed to determine the levels of two substances, lecithin and spingomyelin. When the L/S ratio indicates that the lungs are mature enough, treatment for premature labor may be halted.

An obstetrician may also suggest the use of corticosteroids to promote maturation of the lungs. Use of steroids reduces by half the incidence of hyaline membrane disease (HMD), but this type of treatment is not widespread and has restricted usage based upon gestational age and imminence of delivery. Since steroids have been used for this purpose in the United States only since the mid-1970s, doctors and researchers do not yet know if there are any long-term consequences for infants whose mothers are given steroids. The ability to prevent HMD is a significant breakthrough, however, because HMD is frequently associated with other complications of prematurity.

COPING WITH SUBSEQUENT PREGNANCIES

With any subsequent delivery, even minor problems may be magnified by past experiences. To leave a new baby in the hospital for even one day because of slight jaundice or some other relatively common medical problem is a horrifying thought to many parents who previously have endured weeks or months of separation from a prematurely born infant. Individual responses to subsequent deliveries vary but one mother stated the overriding sentiment of many couples:

> There is always a chance factor to life—and that is what most of us who have had a premie will always have to deal with.

For a woman who has had difficult pregnancies, feelings may be mixed.

In the course of my childbearing attempts, I have had, in order, a miscarriage at around four to five weeks, a premature birth at thirty weeks, a miscarriage at twenty weeks—in spite of having a McDonald stitch—and a miscarriage at eight weeks. The only thing I have yet to experience is a term birth.

If there is a fine line between being foolish and being determined, then I must be walking it, for I have a lot of faith that medical science can pull me through a term birth yet.

Every time I have become pregnant, I have greeted the news with the attitude that we'll take what comes and we'll make it. Well, it gets harder and harder to do that because I have a tendency to lump all the bad experiences together.

I don't actually sit around and say, "Oh, I'll never make it with this one either," but I do wonder what the outcome will be. I wish that I could throw myself joyfully into each pregnancy, but instead I've built a wall around me that makes euphoria hard to come by.

And so I wait once again for another "next time." My husband waits with me—loving, confident and full of positive thoughts. My son waits, too, although he's too young to know it. He shows me daily why I want to keep trying and makes me realize how much I have already been blessed.

Fears and worries are inescapable during future pregnancies. Concerns may be of a personal nature or related solely to the health of the unborn child.

My obstetrician told me in my fourth month of pregnancy that I would have to quit work if I had any contractions at all. I spent months terrified that I could lose a very new and enjoyable career and yet still could face the possibility of losing a premie, too.

Journal entry: March 29—Baby is a dancer, a mover. No waltzes, just primitive rhythms and drums—a baby whale surfacing into the sun—delighted with movement

—seeking the elements—a creature of the water, breathing air.

You are always telling me, "I'm alive, alive, alive." And I'm always whispering, "Stay a little longer—please wait until you're ready—spare yourself the pain of prematurity."

Eleven weeks until my due date. Already my bag for the hospital is semipacked—already the mental preparations, just in case. Yes, I worry. I mark each day off the four calendars throughout our house. I look at pictures of babies at your stage of development and shudder at the percentages. Don't be born now. Wait.

SUGGESTIONS FOR A CONFINED MOTHER-TO-BE

Bed rest may be a necessity with a high-risk pregnancy. If a mother expects to be in bed for days or weeks, the following checklist may be helpful:

1. If your doctor advises you to discontinue sexual intercourse until your baby is born, be sure you understand the implications. This may include any stimulation that would bring the woman to orgasm, since orgasm could trigger contractions. Discuss sexual questions frankly with your doctor or ask his nurse to find out for you.

2. If you think you are in labor, do not wait; call your doctor or go immediately to the hospital. If an unfamiliar doctor or nurse returns your call, be sure to explain to them your past pregnancy complications. Sometimes getting to the hospital early can give you and your baby valuable time if labor can be halted.

3. Since you may be restricted from physical activity during pregnancy, try to be in your best physical shape before becoming pregnant. After you are pregnant, be conscious of excessive weight gain. If exercise is restricted, you gain quickly. Fresh fruits and vegetables and whole-grain breads and cereals will help regulate sluggish bowels while you are inactive. Sitting and reclining for weeks can also lead to pain-

ful leg cramps. Keep your legs elevated and ask someone to massage them occasionally.

4. If you have to cough or sneeze, slightly tense the pelvic muscles beforehand. Use the same muscles you would use to stop the flow of urine. This is a protective measure taught in Lamaze classes. It is especially important in a high-risk pregnancy.

5. Look on the positive side. Enjoy the rest and relaxation. It may seem like you will be restricted "forever," but it is only several months or weeks out of the rest of your life. This is your first contribution to caring for your baby. If you are feeling depressed, call someone who has been through similar circumstances.

6. Shop around for a good housecleaning service. For a few hours once a week, let someone else tackle the most difficult chores of housekeeping.

7. The care of your children may be shared by relatives, friends and schools. Make notes for those helping you. Give them a list of telephone numbers; directions to the pediatrician's office; an outline of your child's food preferences, medications and daily routine; and a list of items you will need in the hospital and where to locate them.

8. You can still be an active mother while in bed. Have on hand books, games or learning cards for your children. (A teacher's supply store is loaded with goodies!) Put together a crafts box of crayons, scissors, paper, etc. Let children assist you when possible. If children understand that mommy must stay in bed, they may find satisfaction in helping.

9. Consider your personal likes and comforts. You will need a telephone nearby. You may also need extra pillows. A rolling cart is handy for meals, water, cosmetics and any extras you may need. Magazines, books, a piece of needlework or some other craft can be enjoyed in bed. You can write letters, design birth announcements, even make Christmas decorations or presents. Keep a journal about your feelings if you like. Put your photograph album or recipe file in order.

10. You need not live in a nightgown or uncomfortable

clothing while restricted. Since there may be visitors, helpers and others in and out of your hourse for a while, consider comfortable, easy-care housedresses. Front buttons or zippers make nursing or pumping more convenient after the baby is born.

11. If friends, neighbors or relatives offer to help, say yes! Let others share their caring for you and your family. It is often easier for people to be useful if they know how to help. Suggest they do one particular chore for you:

a. Make one meal to put in the freezer.

b. Buy groceries for a week.

c. Do one day's laundry.

d. Baby-sit for one afternoon; take your children for an outing.

e. Water plants and lawn.

f. Prepare a tray of healthful snacks for you and your children.

g. Shop for personal items.

Most of all, let your friends know that you need their support and encouragement. Do not hesitate to tell them when you need to talk. Later there will be time for you to repay kindnesses. Meanwhile, you have given a lot of people the satisfaction of helping you move closer to delivering a healthy baby.

THE NEXT TIMES

Women with high-risk histories may have repeatedly disappointing pregnancies, but as medical technology and techniques improve, many couples can anticipate better outcomes of pregnancy. For some, a premature birth is simply an accident of nature that may not recur.

Many of the children mentioned in this book have healthy younger brothers and sisters as a result of better "next times":

• Bryan, born at 3 pounds 3 ounces, ten weeks early, has twin brothers, Tyler and Graham who were born weighing 6 pounds 8 ounces and 7 pounds 3½ ounces respectively, at thirty-seven weeks.

- Chris and Duncan, born at 3 pounds 6½ ounces and 4 pounds 4 ounces respectively, eight weeks early, have a brother, Nicholas, who was born weighing 8 pounds 5 ounces at full term.
- Jennie, born at 3 pounds 7 ounces, seven weeks early (and delivered in the car by her father!), has a brother, Graham, who was born weighing 7 pounds 3 ounces at thirty-six weeks.
- Jennifer, born at 2 pounds 10 ounces, ten weeks early, has a brother, Matthew, who was born weighing 4 pounds 7 ounces at thirty-seven weeks.
- Johanna and Suzanne, born at 2 pounds 2 ounces each, twelve weeks early, have a sister Elizabeth, who was born weighing 6 pounds 7½ ounces on her due date.
- Michael, born at 4 pounds 11 ounces, eight weeks early, has a sister, Suzanne, who was born weighing 8 pounds 1½ ounces at thirty-seven weeks.
- Mindy, born at 2 pounds 3 ounces, thirteen weeks early, has a brother, Dennis, who was born weighing 7 pounds 8 ounces at thirty-eight weeks.
- Monica, born at 2 pounds 9 ounces, ten weeks early, has a brother, Jonathan, who was born weighing 7 pounds 15 ounces at thirty-six weeks.
- Zachary, born at 4 pounds 1 ounce, eight weeks early, has a brother, Jeffrey, born weighing 8 pounds 1 ounce at thirty-seven weeks.

Some of the mothers of these children were confined to bed for a time during pregnancy, had surgery to hold the cervix closed or took other precautions suggested by their doctors. Others did not; but all were careful to consult with their obstetricians often.

The parents of these children can say with one mother:

> What a joy this new little life has been to our home. Our children are so special to us. We realize how very lucky we are to have had them at all. Thanks to modern technology, dedicated doctors (especially my obstetrician) and a superior Being, we have beautiful children.

Parents with better "next times" are granted two special gifts: having a healthy baby and a means of putting the event of prematurity in perspective.

While it is, of course, best not to compare children to one another, comparisons are almost inevitable for parents who have cared for a premature baby and a term baby. Such comparisons can provide positive insights.

> I feel so vindicated now. There is such a difference between this full-term baby and the twins. They were my first so I didn't realize how many of the problems we had with them were due to their prematurity.
>
> I thought I was at fault for the twins' fussiness and not sleeping well. I kept searching every parenting book I could find for answers.
>
> If the twins had a shot or bumped their heads, they cried hysterically. My attempts to comfort them had no effect, and I felt rejected and inept. This baby also cries, but he stops soon after he is picked up.
>
> Our twins cried differently, too. Theirs was a shrill, demanding, incessant cry, and it was constant. This baby wakes up with what I call a casual cry, as if he's saying, "O.K., I'm awake now and would like breakfast." As soon as he sees us he stops crying, waiting expectantly.
>
> This baby amuses himself with anything—wallpaper, shoes, cookie cutters. The twins' attention span was so short. This baby does everything on his own; the twins required our involvement on everything. We were exhausted, mentally and physically.
>
> As I look back now, four years after the twins' birth, I can see how so many problems then and now are related to their inability or delay in integrating their responses to their environment. I am constantly amazed at just how different a full-term baby is.
>
> I'm also ashamed of myself for listening to "well-meaning" relatives and friends who constantly criticized our kids because they expected them to be just like "normal" kids. I expected a slowness in physical development but never realized how all-inclusive the differences would be.
>
> I am convinced that no one can understand what I am

saying except another parent of a premature baby. I have stopped trying to educate the misinformed. The most I can hope for is recognition of the fact that my twins are unique, with their own individual criteria for success.

Do parents of premies ever feel that the problems of prematurity are over? Probably not. The best that parents can do is to place a difficult chapter of their lives in perspective and continue to meet the challenges of raising their unique children.

Appendix 1

GLOSSARY

Acidosis: High acidity of the blood.

Acute fetal distress: See hypoxia.

Alpha-fetoprotein (AFP):   See neural tube defects.

Amnionitis: Infected amniotic fluid.

Anemia: Deficiency of red blood cells, which carry oxygen in the blood to all parts of the body.

Anoxia: Oxygen deprivation.

Antepartum: Before labor.

Apgar score: Assessment of newborn health based on heart rate, respiratory effort, muscle tone, reflex irritability and color.

Apnea: Absence of breathing for more than ten seconds.

Appropriate for gestational age (AGA):   See small for gestational age.

Aspiration: Inhalation into the windpipe and lungs of material such as formula, meconium or stomach juices. Also, the removal of fluids or gases from a body cavity by suction.

Aspiration pneumonia: Pneumonia caused by inhaling foreign substances such as the inhalation of meconium during fetal distress.

Bagging: Pumping air or oxygen into the lungs by means of squeezing an ambu bag into a mask placed over the baby's nose and mouth.

Bilirubin: A pigment in the blood stream that comes from breakdown of the red blood cells and can cause jaundice if the level is too high. The liver usually rids the body of bilirubin.

Blood-gas test: Measurement of gases, such as oxygen, present in the blood.

264

Bradycardia (brachycardia):   Slower than normal heart rate.

Brazelton assessment: Set of criteria used to assess the social behavior of the newborn.

Bronchopulmonary dysplasia (BPD):   Also known as chronic lung disease. Scarring of the lung tissue resulting in breathing difficulty. BPD can occur when infants have been on a respirator for an extended time.

Cerebral palsy (CP):   The aftereffects of damage to the brain during gestation or birth, CP is a nonprogressive disorder of coordination and movement.

Cerebrospinal fluid (CSF):   See spinal tap.

Chest tubes: Tubes placed in the chest to remove trapped air or fluid. Used in the case of a pneumothorax to remove unwanted air and allow the lungs to expand.

Chronic lung disease: See bronchopulmonary dysplasia.

Colic: Excessive crying and drawing-up of the legs in a young baby. May be caused by immature nervous and digestive systems. Colic usually occurs two to four weeks after the due date of the baby.

Collapsed lung: See pneumothorax.

Colostrum: Yellowish fluid (premilk) secreted before and for a few days after the birth of a baby.

Congenital anomalies: Birth defects.

CPAP (continuous positive airway pressure):   A setting on a respirator. Positive pressure applied to the lungs during spontaneous breathing to prevent collapse of the alveoli and air passages during exhalation.

Crib death: See sudden infant death syndrome.

Cupping and clapping: Physical application of a series of taps or claps in the chest area to loosen mucus in the bronchial tubes.

Cyanosis: Bluish discoloration of the skin and lips due to poor circulation or low oxygen concentration in the blood.

Diarrhea, chronic: Chronic diarrhea of unknown cause is also known as chronic nonspecific infant intestinal disorder. It is usually indicative of an immature gastrointestinal system; maturity generally resolves the problem.

Dubowitz assessment: Set of criteria used to assess the gestational age of a newborn.

Eclampsia: Advanced stage of toxemia characterized by convulsions and coma. See also toxemia.

Edema: Excessive accumulation of fluid in body tissues; swelling.

Electrolytes: Certain chemicals in the blood, including sodium, potassium and chloride, that must be present in normal concentrations for optimum function of all body cells.

Endotracheal tube: Small tube which, when placed in the windpipe, delivers air directly to the lungs; may be attached to a respirator.

Erythroblastosis fetalis: See Rh negativity.

Exchange transfusion: Replacement of 70 to 80 percent of circulating blood by withdrawing the recipient's blood and injecting a donor's blood in equal amounts.

Extubation: Removal of the respirator's plastic tubing from the baby's windpipe.

Fetoprotein test: See neural tube defects.

Fetoscope: Special stethoscope used to hear the fetal heartbeat through the mother's abdomen. An amplifying fetoscope conveys sound into the room.

FLK (funny-looking kid):   Term used to alert doctors that there may or may not be other specific problems.

Galactosemia: Hereditary lack of the enzyme necessary to break down milk sugars (lactose, galactose).

Gestation: Period of time from conception to birth. Gestational age is the number of completed weeks in the pregnancy counting from the first day of the last normal menstrual cycle.

Head bleed: See intraventricular hemorrhage.

Hematoma: Collection of blood that clots within tissue to form a solid mass; bruise.

Hemolytic diseases of the newborn: Diseases in which red blood cells are destroyed, resulting in the diffusion throughout the body of breakdown products of hemoglobin (such as bilirubin) which are especially poisonous to brain cells.

Hemorrhagic disease of the newborn: See vitamin K.

Hernia: Protrusion of an organ or part of an organ through a weak spot in surrounding tissue. Umbilical hernia is a protrusion of the bowel through a defect in the abdominal wall.

Hyaline membrane disease (HMD):   Also known as respiratory distress syndrome (RDS) and as idiopathic respiratory syndrome. HMD is caused by a lack of pulmonary surfactant, a substance that affects the surface tension of the alveoli, or tiny air sacs, within the lungs. Without enough surfactant, the alveoli collapse and fail to expand. As a result, oxygen levels in the blood become low and the baby's breathing becomes difficult.

Hydrocephalus: Excessive accumulation of cerebrospinal fluid within the ventricles of the brain caused by blockage of the normal circulation or malabsorption.

Hyperalimentation: Administration of nutrients by IV to a baby who cannot be fed by mouth for some reason.

Hyperbilirubinemia: An excess of bilirubin in the blood. See also jaundice.

Hypertension: High blood pressure.

Hyperthyroidism: Excessive secretion of thyroid hormone.

Hypocalcemia: Below normal level of calcium in the blood.

Hypoglycemia: Abnormally small concentration of sugar in the blood.

Hypotension: Abnormally low blood pressure.

Hypothyroidism: Undersecretion of the thyroid hormone.

Hypoxia: Also called acute fetal distress; occurs when the fetus is not getting adequate oxygen.

Incubator: An enclosed environment providing warmth, oxygen and a fairly germ-free atmosphere for the newborn.

Inhalation therapy: Administration by inhalation of a medicinal mist, sometimes combined with oxygen that loosens mucus in the bronchial tubes.

Intercranial hemorrhage (ICH):   Bleeding within the skull or cranium.

Interstitial emphysema: Pockets of air in the lungs. Occurs while on a respirator when the high pressure forces air into the alveoli.

Intraventricular hemorrhage (IVH):   Bleeding within the ventricles of the brain; sometimes called a head bleed.

Intubation: Placing a small plastic tube through the nose or mouth into the baby's windpipe to assist breathing or into the esophagus for feeding.

IPPB (intermittent positive pressure breathing):   Inflating the lungs during inspiration by positive pressure from a machine.

Jaundice: Yellow discoloration of the body tissues caused by the deposit of bile pigments (bilirubin). Physiologic jaundice is that which occurs in an otherwise healthy newborn more than twenty-four to thirty-six hours of age. Any jaundice that is not physiologic is pathologic. Breast-milk jaundice occurs when a substance in breast milk (pregnanediol) inhibits the breakdown of bilirubin by interfering with an enzyme in the infant's body. The infant's ability to break down pregnanediol and thus, bilirubin, increases with maturity, and jaundice subsides.

Lactation: Secretion of breast milk.

Lactose intolerance: Inability to break down lactose, a sugar that is found in human milk and cow's milk.

Large for gestational age (LGA):   See small for gestational age.

Lumbar puncture: See spinal tap.

Meconium: First stools of an infant; thick, sticky and dark greenish brown.

Meconium staining: Discoloration caused when meconium is expelled into the amniotic fluid by the fetus.

Metabolic toxemia of late pregnancy (MTLP):   See toxemia.

Milk bank: Facility that collects and stores breast milk from a variety of mothers for research purposes and/or for distribution to infants whose mothers cannot supply breast milk.

Minimal brain dysfunction (MBD):   Mild brain damage that may lead to learning disabilities, hyperactivity, slight gross- and fine-motor control problems, etc.

Necrotizing enterocolitis (NEC):   Inflammatory disease of the stomach-intestinal tract, frequently complicated by perforation.

Neural tube defects: Birth defects of the brain and/or spinal cord such as spina bifida and anencephaly. Neural tube defects may be detected in utero with the fetoprotein test which measures the amount of alpha-fetoprotein, the major circulating protein of the human fetus, in amniotic fluid.

Patent ductus arteriosus (PDA, open ductus, patent ductus):   An anatomic connection between the lungs and heart, the ductus arteriosus is usually open during fetal life but normally closes shortly prior to or after birth.

PEEP (positive end expiratory pressure):   A method used in conjunction with a ventilator in the treatment of respiratory distress. Applies continuous pressure to the lungs to prevent alveolar collapse during expiration.

Perinatologist: An obstetrician who deals primarily with high-risk mothers and infants, especially during the perinatal period, that is, the time just prior to and up to about four weeks after birth.

Perinatology: The branch of medicine dealing with care of the new-born and mother up to about four weeks after birth.

Periodic breathing: Brief apnea spells without cyanosis; common in the respiration of premature infants.

Persistent fetal circulation (PFC):   Condition in which the blood circulation in a newborn continues to flow as in the fetus. Normally, there are changes in blood circulation after birth that enable the newborn to function better on its own.

PKU (phenylketonuria):   Enzyme deficiency causing inability to digest protein.

Placental insufficiency: Condition in which the placenta does not function as it should.

Pneumothorax: Collapse of a lung. After this occurs, air is found in the thoracic cavity surrounding the lungs.

Polycythemia: An excess of red blood cells in the blood.

Postural drainage (chest):   A procedure which places a patient in a dyundent position allowing secretions to drain from air passageways by gravity.

Preeclampsia: The first stage of toxemia, characterized by swelling, high blood pressure and the presence of albumin in the urine. See also toxemia.

Pulmonary oxygen toxicity (POT):   See bronchopulmonary dysplasia.

Respiration therapy: See inhalation therapy.

Respirator: A machine that assists in breathing by regulating the flow of air into and out of the lungs. Same as ventilator.

Respiratory distress: Fast or labored breathing. More severe cases are termed respiratory distress syndrome or hyaline membrane disease.

Respiratory distress syndrome (RDS):   See hyaline membrane disease.

Retinopathy of prematurity: Abnormal condition of the retina found in some premature infants.

Retracting: "Caving in" of the chest as the baby breathes; a common symptom of respiratory distress.

Retrolental fibroplasia (RLF):   Condition characterized by the formation of an opaque tissue behind the lens of the eye that is caused by a too high concentration of oxygen given to an immature infant. May lead to interrupted growth of the eye or detachment of the retina.

Rh negativity: When the mother's blood lacks the Rh factor (Rh negative) and the fetus has the factor (Rh positive), the mother's body may treat the fetus as a foreign substance and manufacture antibodies which attack the fetus. Rh disease (erythroblastosis fetalis) occurs when the mother's sensitized immune system crosses the placenta and attacks the fetal red blood cells.

Room air: Normal room air has an oxygen concentration of approximately 21 percent.

Rooting reflex: Instinctive response of a newborn to seek out the nipple when touched on or around the cheek.

Sepsis: An infection of the blood stream or tissues.

Shake test: Test to assess amniotic fluid to determine lung maturity in the fetus; faster and simpler than the L/S ratio test.

Shunt: Plastic tube leading from a blocked ventricle of the brain (in hydrocephalus) to drain fluid to the heart or abdominal area.

Small for gestational age (SGA):   Infant whose birth weight is below the tenth percentile. Appropriate for gestational age (AGA) includes birth weights between the tenth and ninetieth percentiles. Large for gestational age (LGA) is over the ninetieth percentile.

Spinal tap: Withdrawal of a small amount of the cerebrospinal fluid (CSF) contained in the brain and spinal cord for analysis. A lumbar puncture is a spinal tap of the lower spinal column.

Standing orders: Doctor's "blanket instructions" for routine use of medicines and procedures to be given to his patients during his absence.

Stress test: Administration of labor-stimulating drugs in small quantities to assess fetal stress under labor conditions prior to actual labor.

Sucking reflex: Instinctive response of a newborn when stimulated around the lips to use the mouth and jaws.

Suction: Procedure to remove mucus and secretions from the nose, throat or endotracheal tube using a small plastic tube attached to a vacuum.

Sudden infant death syndrome (SIDS):   Also known as crib death. Condition of unknown cause in which an apparently healthy baby dies suddenly and unexpectedly, usually while sleeping.

Surfactant: See hyaline membrane disease, respiratory distress syndrome.

Toxemia: Disorder occurring during pregnancy or shortly after delivery that is characterized by one or all of the following: swelling, high blood pressure, presence of albumin in the urine, convulsions and coma. Metabolic toxemia of late pregnancy is considered to be a complication caused by inadequate diet or malnutrition. See also preeclampsia, eclampsia.

Transient tachypnea of the newborn: Rapid breathing for several days after birth due to fluid in the lungs that clears by itself as fluid is absorbed.

Ventilation: Administration of air with varying levels of oxygen through a ventilator or respirator.

Vitamin E: Thought to help prevent a condition causing blindness (retrolental fibroplasia)

Vitamin K: Often given by injection soon after birth to prevent a bleeding disorder, called hemorrhagic disease of the newborn, caused by vitamin K deficiency. Premature infants are usually deficient in vitamin K.

Appendix 2

RESOURCES*

SUGGESTED READING

There are many excellent publications, in addition to those listed, on the following topics. The books, pamphlets and articles suggested for further reading are ones that other parents of premature infants and leaders of parent support groups have found useful.

A special section recommends books and articles that may be of interest to neonatology professionals or others in the medical field. Parents would be well advised not to attempt to locate and read neonatology textbooks because the information in them is generally so technical that it is confusing to those with no medical training. In addition, advances in neonatology occur so rapidly that the information in textbooks is quickly outdated.

Childbearing and Prematurity

> Galinsky, Ellen. *Beginnings: A Young Mother's Personal Account of Two Premature Births.* Boston: Houghton Mifflin, 1976.

272

Langhurst, M. Jude, B.A. *"My Baby Is a Special Care Infant: A Parent's Guide to Neonatal Intensive Care."* Wichita, Kansas: Parents and Friends of Special Care Infants, 1981. Available from PFSCI, 1452 Melrose, Wichita, Kansas 67212.

Leach, Penelope. *Your Baby and Child: From Birth to Age Five.* New York: Alfred A. Knopf, 1978.

Metcalf, Sharon Cozine. *Getting to Know Your Premature Baby.* Louisville, Kentucky: University of Louisville, 1978. Available from S. C. Metcalf, R.N., M.S.W., Children and Youth Project, Department of Pediatrics, University of Louisville, 323 E. Chestnut Street, Louisville, Kentucky 40203.

National Institute of Mental Health, U.S. Department of Health and Human Services. *Pre-Term Babies.* Washington, D.C., 1980. U.S. Government Printing Office, Superintendent of Documents, Washington, D.C. 20402. A pamphlet in the Caring About Kids series. Other pamphlets discuss hyperactivity, dyslexia and related topics.

Shosenberg, Nancy. *The Premature Infant: A Handbook for Parents.* Toronto, Ontario: The Hospital for Sick Children, 1980. Available from The Hospital for Sick Children, Room 1218, 555 University Avenue, Toronto, Ontario, Canada MSG1x8.

Special Hospital Care for Your New Baby. Columbus, Ohio: Ross Laboratories, 1978. Available in many NICUs or from Ross Laboratories, 625 Cleveland, Columbus, Ohio 43216.

Hospitals

Bell, David. *A Time to Be Born.* New York: William Morrow, 1975.

Colen, B.D. *Born at Risk.* New York: St. Martin's, 1981.

Gots, Ronald and Kaufman, Arthur. *The People's Hospital Book.* New York: Crown, 1978.

Marriage

Lederer, William J., and Jackson, Don D. *The Mirages of Marriage.* New York: W.W. Norton, 1968.

Infant Care and Development

Brazelton, T. Berry. *On Becoming a Family.* New York: Delacorte, 1981.

Burck, Frances Wells. *Babysense.* New York: St. Martin's, 1979.

Caplan, Frank, ed., Princeton Center for Infancy. *The Parenting Advisor.* Garden City, New York: Anchor Press, 1977.

Green, Martin I., ed. *A Sigh of Relief: The First-Aid Handbook for Childhood Emergencies.* New York: Bantam Books, 1977.

Massachusetts Department of Mental Health. *Home Stimulation for the Young Developmentally Disabled Child (1973)* and *Exploring Materials With Your Young Child With Special Needs (1974).* Boston: Media Resource Center, Massachusetts Department of Mental Health. Available from Commonwealth Mental Health Foundation, 4 Marlboro Road, Lexington, Massachusetts 02173.

White, Burton L. *the First Three Years of Life.* Englewood Cliffs, New Jersey: Prentice-Hall, 1975. Also available is the *Parent's Guide to the First Three Years of Life.*

Parenting

Biller, Henry and Meredith, Dennis. *Father Power.* New York: David McKay, 1974.

Dodson, Fitzhugh. *How to Parent.* Los Angeles: Nash, 1970.

Dreikurs, Rudolf with Soltz, Vicki. *Children: The Challenge.* New York: Hawthorn, 1964.

The Free Stuff Editors. *Free Stuff for Parents.* Deephaven, Minnesota: Meadowbrook Press, 1980. Also sold by Meadowbrook Press are three books of lighthearted cartoons about pregnancy, birth and raising children. All are by Lynn Johnson—*David, We're Pregnant, Hi Mom! Hi Dad!* and *Do They Ever Grow Up?*—and are great tension relievers.

Galinsky, Ellen. Between Generations: *The Six Stages of Parenthood.* New York: Times Books, 1981.

Gordon, Thomas. *P.E.T. Parent Effectiveness Training: The Tested New Way to Raise Responsible Children.* New York: The New American Library, 1975.

Breast-Feeding

Brewster, Dorothy Patricia. *You Can Breastfeed Your Baby . . . Even in Special Situations.* Emmaus, Pennsylvania: Rodale Press, 1979.

Eiger, Marvin S., and Olds, Sally Wendkos. *The Complete Book of Breastfeeding.* New York: Workman, Bantam Books, 1972.

Ewy, Donna and Ewy, Rodger. *Preparation for Breastfeeding.* New York: Doubleday, 1975.

Hill, Reba Michels. *"A Passage in Life: Breast Feeding."* 1978. Available from Parents of Prematures, c/o HOPE, 3311 Richmond, Suite 330, Houston, Texas 77098.

La Leche League International, Inc. *The New Womanly Art of Breastfeeding.* Franklin Park, Illinois: La Leche League International, 1981. Also available is "Breastfeeding Your Premature Baby," 1980.

Coping With Emotions, Death and Dying

Borg, Susan and Lasker, Judith. *When Pregnancy Fails: Families Coping with Miscarriage, Stillbirth and Infant Death.* Boston: Beacon Press, 1981.

DelliQuadri, Lyn and Breckenridge, Kati. *Mother Care: Helping Yourself Through the Emotional and Physical Transitions of New Motherhood.* Los Angeles: J.P. Tarcher, n.d.

Editors of *Consumer Reports. Funerals: Consumers' Last Rights.* New York: W.W. Norton, 1977.

My Baby Died . . . Ways to Cope with the Death of a Newborn. Westmont, Illinois: Parenting Publications, n.d. Available from Parenting Publications, P.O. Box 98, Westmont, Illinois 60559.

Peppers, Larry G. and Knapp, Ronald J. *Motherhood and Mourning: Perinatal Death.* New York: Praeger Publishers, 1980.

Schift, Harriet. *The Bereaved Parent.* New York: Crown, 1977.

Wolf, Anna W.M. *Helping Your Child to Understand Death.* New York: Child Study Press, 1973.

Recommended for Professionals

Goldberg, Susan. "Premature Birth: Consequences for the Parent-Infant Relationship." *American Scientist* March–April 1979, vol. 67, no. 2, 214–220.

Kane, Leslie. "Critically Ill Newborns: Should the Health Care Team Include Parents?" *St. Joseph Hospital Medical Journal* 13 (1978): 225–229. Available from

St. Joseph's Hospital, 1919 LaBranch, Houston, Texas 77002.

Moore, Mary Lou. *Realities in Childbearing.* Philadelphia: W.B. Saunders, 1978.

Noland, Robert L., ed. *Counseling Parents of the Ill and the Handicapped.* Springfield, Illinois: Charles C. Thomas, 1971.

Schwartz, Jane L. and Schwartz, Lawrence H., eds. *Vulnerable Infants: A Psychosocial Dilemma.* New York: McGraw-Hill, 1977.

Wallens, Patricia B.; Elder, Wanda B.; and Hastings, Susan N. *From the Beginning: The EMI High Risk Nursery Intervention Program Manual.* Charlottesville, Virginia: Education for Multihandicapped Infant Project, Available from the Department of Pediatrics, University of Virginia School of Medicine, Box 232, Medical Center, Charlottesville, Virginia 22901.

Self-Help Groups

Ardman, Perri and Ardman, Harvey. *Woman's Day Book of Fund Raising.* New York: St. Martin's Press, 1980.

Armstrong, Julie; Edmondson, Judy; Honikman, Jane; and Mrstik, Judy. *A Guide for Establishing a Parent Support Program in Your Community.* Santa Barbara, California: Postpartum Education for Parents (PEP), Inc., 1979. Available from PEP, Inc., 927 N. Kellog Avenue Santa Barbara, California 98111.

Connors, Tracy D., ed. *The Nonprofit Organization Handbook.* New York: McGraw-Hill, 1980.

Mason, Diane; Jensen, Gayle; and Ryzewicz, Carolyn. *How to Grow a Parent's Group.* Milwaukee, Wisconsin: International Childbirth Education Association, 1979. Available from ICEA Bookstore or CDG Enterprises, P.O. Box 97, Western Springs, Illinois 60558.

PARENTING MAGAZINES AND NEWSLETTERS

In addition to the many books now available on parenting, there are a number of magazines and newsletters that focus on ways parents can do an effective job in raising healthy, happy children. They offer sample issues free or for a slight charge.

The following list includes a few of these publications that parents have found helpful. Other, better known magazines and newsletters have been omitted here, because parents can find information on them in other source books.

Building Blocks
314 Liberty
Box 31
Dundee, Illinois 60118

The Exceptional Parent
296 Boylston Street
Third Floor
Boston, Massachusetts 02116

Mothering
P.O. Box 2046
Albuquerque, New Mexico 87103

Pediatrics for Parents: The Monthly Newsletter for Caring Parents
Box 1069
Bangor, Maine 04401

Practical Parenting
18318 Minnetonka Boulevard
Deephaven, Minnesota 55391

BOOK CATALOGS AND OTHER SOURCES

In some communities, it may be difficult to locate the books listed here or others on the various topics. Most bookstores will place orders for their customers, and in some cities, there are bookstores that specialize in books on childbirth, infant care and development and parenting. Government publications may be ordered from the U.S. Government Printing Office in Washington or purchased at GPO bookstores located in various cities across the country. Single copies of some government publications are often free from the agency that prepared the publication.

The following specialized bookstores offer mail-order service for book buyers:

Birth & Life Bookstore
P.O. Box 70625
Seattle, Washington 98107

ICEA Bookcenter
P.O. Box 20048
Minneapolis, Minnesota 55420

The Orange Cat
442 Church Street
Garberville, California 95440

U.S. Government Printing Office
Superintendent of Documents
Washington, D.C. 20402

CLOTHES

Ready-to-wear lines for premies are available nationally or in selected regions of the country. Those marked with an asterisk have catalogs available and offer garments by mail.

Many of the manufacturers listed offer only a limited line of premie-size items. If parents cannot find premie fashions in their area, they may wish to order garments from those businesses that sell by mail or to ask local retail stores to contact wholesalers to obtain clothing for resale.

*Anne's Preemie Wear
c/o Anne Long

Route 12, Fairview Drive
Greenville, South Carolina 29609

Baby Bliss
227 Spring Street
Middleville, Michigan 48333

Isaacson-Carrico
P.O. Box 1060
El Campo, Texas 77437

*Lilletot by Judy C. Mickelsen
1880 Coronada Drive
Ann Arbor, Michigan 48103

*Oh So Small
Joanne Bock
6432 Pacific Avenue
Tacoma, Washington 98408

Paty, Inc.
4800 West 34th, Suite A-9
Houston, Texas 77092

*Pee Wee Creations
Deborah Dean
7809 W. Bellfort #104
Houston, Texas 77071

The Pine Nuts
P.O. Box 559
Airway Heights, Washington 99001

*Premie Petites
Francis & Associates
Manufacturers Representatives
3318 Western #117
Amarillo, Texas 79109

Premiers by Alexis
Warren Featherbone Co.
P.O. Box 383
Gainesville, Georgia 30501

Shirey, Inc.
1017 Stanford
Greenville, Texas 75401

S. Schwab Co., Inc.
P.O. Box 1417
Cumberland, Maryland 21502

Tic Toc Infants Wear
P.O. Box 787
Brenham, Texas 77833

*Tiny Mite Premie Fashions
Janet Thayer, R.N.
P.O. Box 6346
Glendale, California 91205

Toddle Tyke
440 Armour Place
Atlanta, Georgia 30324

Too Small
4822 Lido Lane
Houston, Texas 77092

Zona Lee
986 Mission Street
San Francisco, California 94103

DIAPERS

Premie Pampers (TM) are available from the manufacturer, Proctor and Gamble. Sold only by the case (180 diapers), premie-size Pampers fit babies up to 6 pounds. To order, call toll free 1-800-543-4932. Use Visa or Mastercard, or pay COD charges.

Some local pharmacies or hospitals may special order Premie Pampers.

Newborn-size disposable diapers may be cut to the appropriate size and retaped with masking tape.

Regular cloth diapers may also be cut in half for use with a small baby. A specially shaped cloth diaper, the Dexter B-29, may be adjusted by folding in side flaps to fit a premie. Dexter B-29s are available by mail from:

Dexter Diaper Factory
236 W. 17th Street

P.O. Box 7367

Houston, Texas 77008

Premie-size cloth diapers made of six layers of topstitched flannel are available from:

Premie Pals Custom Fitted Diapers
Nancy Nelson
1313 Harrington Avenue S.E.
Renton, Washington 98055

Plastic pants are made by Premiers by Alexis and plastic-lined fabric diaper covers are made by Premie Petites (see Clothing section).

BREAST PUMPING AND NURSING

Write manufacturers for information or names and addresses of local distributors. To locate a pump, contact the local chapter of La Leche League (LLL), the nursery staff, your obstetrician, support groups for parents, childbirth education organizations or medical supply rental businesses. Hospitals may have pumps available for short-term or in-hospital use.

Hand Pumps

Kaneson Breast Milking/Feeding Unit
Happy Family Products
1251 S. La Cienega Boulevard
Los Angeles, California 90035

Loyd-B Pump
LOPUCO
1615 Old Annapolis Road
Woodbine, Maryland 21797

Ora'lac Pump
Box 137
Sitka, Alaska 99835

Rubber bulb suction pumps are available at local pharmacies.

Electric Pumps

Egnell, Inc.
412 Park Avenue
Cary, Illinois 60013

GOMCO
828 E. Ferry Street
Buffalo, New York 14211

Medela, Inc.
457 Dartmoor Drive
P.O. Box 386
Crystal Lake, Illinois 60014

Lact-Aid

The Lact-Aid nursing supplementer may be obtained from some LLL chapters. It also may be rented or purchased from:

Resources in Human Nurturing International
Lact-Aid and Service Supply Center
Box 6861
Denver, Colorado 80206

J.J. Avery Inc.
P.O. Box 6459
Denver, Colorado 80206

Organizations

For further support and information about breast pumping and nursing contact:

La Leche League
9616 Minneapolis Avenue
Franklin Park, Illinois 60131

Resources in Human Nurturing International (see above)

Counselors

The following is a list of lactation counselors who specialize in providing information on breast-feeding the premature infant. They all present seminars and accept telephone referrals.

Kathleen Auerbach, Ph.D.
Department of Sociology
University of Nebraska at Omaha
Omaha, Nebraska 68182
(402) 554-2632

Bethany Hays, M.D., and Theodora von Furestenberg
Baylor College of Medicine
Lactation Clinic
1200 Moursund
Houston, Texas 77030
(713) 797-0322, twenty-four-hour hotline

Reba Michels Hill, M.D.
Chief of Newborn Research
St. Luke's Episcopal Hospital
720 Bertner
Houston, Texas 77030
(713) 791-3184

Lauri Lowen
President, Parents of Prematures (Seattle)
13613 N.E. 26th Place
Bellevue, Washington 98005
(206) 883-6040

Marianne Neifert, M.D.
Assistant Professor of Pediatrics
University of Colorado School of Medicine
No referrals by mail
(303) 394-7963

SUPPORT GROUPS

For Parents of Premature Infants

In many communities, parents have joined together to support each other and parents of newborn premies in various ways.

Some groups raise funds for hospital nurseries or offer parents practical advice and information. Others have programs of personal contact between new parents and those who have faced a similar situation. The list of activities and projects is as varied as the groups are.

While some support groups are highly structured, with officers, bylaws and established meeting calendars and projects, others are small and conduct business more informally. A particular hospital may sponsor a group, or the group may be community based.

Although each group's specific goals and projects differ, all share the common desire to assist new parents in any way possible as they face the crisis of a premature birth. In order to fulfill this desire, groups must be willing to work with the medical professionals in their community and vice versa. The involvement of doctors, nurses and social workers in the group offers some advantages as well as some disadvantages.

New parents may wish to check first with doctors, nurses or the hospital social worker to ascertain if there is a parent support group in their community.

The following list includes only parent support groups known to Parents of Prematures, Houston Organization for Parent Education, Inc.

This list is for information only; Parents of Prematures does not recommend or endorse any particular group. The list is undoubtedly incomplete, as groups disband or organize frequently. Because of this tendency, no details are given about the groups. For further information, contact the person listed or write to the group:

ARIZONA

Good Samaritan Hospital
Suzanne Wooley
1033 E. McDowell
Phoenix, Arizona 85031
(602) 257-2000

Tucson Parents Group
Harriet Harrell
University of Arizona
Health Services Center
1501 N. Campbell
Tucson, Arizona 85724
(602) 626-6818

CALIFORNIA

Children's Hospital Parents Support Group
Attn: Carolyn Lund, R.N., or Karen Flatley, R.N.
Children's Hospital Medical Center
3200 Telegraph
Oakland, California 94609
(415) 428-3436 or 428-3395

P.S. We Care NICU
University of California at Irvine Medical
Center
101 City Drive S.
Orange, California 92668
*Lynn Clark (714) 963-5393

Parent-to-Parent of Children's Hospital of
San Francisco
3700 California Street
P.O. Box 3805
San Francisco, California 94119

Parent Support Group, A–203
University of California at San Francisco
San Francisco, California 94143

Wee Care
Debby A. Kincaid

1424 S. Parton
Santa Ana, California 92707
(714) 346-6422

COLORADO

Premature Parenthood
c/o Newborn Center
Colorado General Hospital
Box B-195
4200 E. 9th Avenue
Denver, Colorado 80201

Parent-to-Parent of Children's Hospital—
Denver
Cindy Cleveland, R.N.
1056 E. 19th Avenue
Denver, Colorado 80218
(303) 861-6883

St. Mary's ICU Graduate Parent Group
Eloise Barker
2340 Carolina Drive
Grand Junction, Colorado 81503
(303) 245-1338

FLORIDA

Neonatal Parents Support Group, Inc.
Christina Diez
5130 S.W. 114th Court
Miami, Florida 33165
(305) 279-4710

ILLINOIS

Parents Support Group
Kathleen Cull, R.N. and Martina Evans, R.N.
Michael Reese Hospital and Medical Center
29th Street and Ellis Avenue
Chicago, Illinois 60616
(312) 791-4216

Parent-to-Parent Support
Special Care Nursery
Rush-Presbyterian-St. Luke's Medical Center
1753 W. Congress Parkway
Chicago, Illinois 60612

The Will County High-Risk Infant Parent's
Association
Jim Jackson, Chairman
422 Connor
Lockport, Illinois 60441
(815) 838-8891

Southwest Parents Support Group, Inc.
c/o Christ Hospital
4440 W. 95th Street
Oak Lawn, Illinois 60453
(312) 424-8000

Concerned Parents Organization
Lutheran General Hospital
1775 Dempster Street
Park Ridge, Illinois 60068

The Premature and High-Risk Infant
Association
Karen Engel
P.O. Box 3714
Peoria, Illinois 61614

High-Risk Parent Group
Harry Tallackson, Chairman
3616 Prairie Road
Rockford, Illinois 61102

Loyola Premature and High-Risk Infant
Parent's Association
Barb Olenicki
1021 Garner
Wheaton, Illinois 60187
(312) 665-8969

INDIANA

Neo-Fight
Debbie Snyder
130 Red Oak Court
Carmel, Indiana 46032
(317) 844-2212

IOWA

Pilot Parents of Prematures
Bonnie F. Miller
1930 2nd Avenue N.
Fort Dodge, Iowa 50501

KANSAS

Parents and Friends of Special Care Infants
M. Jude Langhurst, President
1452 Melrose
Wichita, Kansas 67212

KENTUCKY

Neo-Life, Inc.
Ginny Foster, President
2201 Azalea Drive
Lexington, Kentucky 40504
(606) 277-5198

LOUISIANA

NICU Parents
Kathie Tobey
1346 Havenwood Drive
Baton Rouge, Louisiana 70815
(504) 275-1590

MASSACHUSETTS

Parent Support Group
Susan Longobucco, R.N.
300 Longwood Avenue
Boston, Massachusetts 02115
(617) 735-7301

MICHIGAN

Support Group for Parents of NICU Babies
Butterworth Hospital
100 Michigan Street N.E.
Grand Rapids, Michigan 49503
(616) 774-1774

MISSOURI

Bonnie Rowley
9909 Kimker Lane
Sunset Hills, Missouri 63127

NEW MEXICO

Action for Newborns
Sherry Curry, President
5605 Bentwood Trail N.E.
Albuquerque, New Mexico 87109
(505) 821-3349

NORTH CAROLINA

Parents Together
Judy Hester
Wake County Medical Center
3000 New Bern Avenue
Raleigh, North Carolina 27610
(919) 755-8545

OHIO

Helping Other Parents Emotionally
Rhonda Richlovsky
1777 Saratoga
Cleveland, Ohio 44109
(216) 398-1642

PENNSYLVANIA

FAMLEE
P.O. Box 15
Telford, Pennsylvania 18969
(215) 257-8554

TEXAS

Graduate Parents
Janet Blalock
P.O. Box 9702
Austin, Texas 78766
(512) 346-5534

Parent Love
Janell Myers
10729 Benbrook
Dallas, Texas 75228
(214) 270-5095

ICN Providence Hospital
Margarita Lozano, R.N.
2001 N. Oregon
El Paso, Texas 79902
(915) 542-6011

Bexar County Parents of Prematures
Pat Falbo
854 E. Sunshine
San Antonio, Texas 78228

Parent-to-Parent, Tarrant County
c/o Cathy Sunkel
2148 Hurstview Drive

Hurst, Texas 76053
(817) 485-0582

Parents of Prematures
c/o Houston Organization for Parent Education,
Inc.
3311 Richmond, Suite 330
Houston, Texas 77098
(713) 524-3089

Golden Crescent Parents of Prematures and High
Risk Infants
Betty Lynch
Route 1, Box 86C
Victoria, Texas 77901
(512) 575-6970

UTAH

Parent-to-Parent
Intermountain Newborn Intensive Care Center
(INICC)
University of Utah Medical Center
50 N. Medical Drive
Salt Lake City, Utah 84132
Sandy Garrand, Family Nurse Consultant
(801) 581-7705

WASHINGTON

Parents of Prematures
Lauri Lowen, President
13613 N.E. 26th Place
Bellevue, Washington 98005
(206) 883-6040

Inland Empire Perinatal Support Group
Elsa C. Distelhorst
W. 1622 Fairway Drive
Spokane, Washington 99218
(509) 466-8287

Robert M. Skarin, M.D.
Neonatal Intensive Care Unit
Madigan Army Medical Center
Tacoma, Washington 98431
(206) 967-6878

WISCONSIN

Diane Barnett
4927 W. Donna Drive
Brown Deer, Wisconsin 98431
(414) 355-7350

CANADA

c/o Social Worker
Special Care Nursery
Children's Hospital
4480 Oak Street
Vancouver, British Columbia, Canada
V6H 3V4

For Bereaved Parents

In addition to the following national organizations, there are a number of local, hospital or community-based groups. If your infant dies, the doctors, nurses or hospital social worker may be helpful in directing you to such groups.

Compassionate Friends
P.O. Box 3247
Hialeah, Florida 33013

National Sudden Infant Death Syndrome
Foundation
310 S. Michigan Avenue, Suite 1904
Chicago, Illinois 60604

For Abusing Parents

> Parents Anonymous
> 2810 Artesia Boulevard, Suite F
> Redondo Beach, California 90278

For Social Workers

> National Association of Perinatal Social
> Workers
> 3311 N. Youngs Boulevard
> Oklahoma City, Oklahoma 73112

Information Sources for Groups

Another source of information on national and local community self-help groups is:

> National Self-help Clearinghouse
> Graduate School and University Center
> City University of New York
> 33 W. 42nd Street, Room 1227
> New York, New York 10036

Nonprofit organizations that offers information and advice on volunteerism is:

> Volunteer: The National Center
> for Citizen Involvement
> P.O. Box 4179
> Boulder, Colorado 80306

HEALTH-RELATED ORGANIZATIONS

Medical professionals, social workers, relatives and friends often encourage parents whose children have long-term medical problems or learning disabilities to contact local or national health-related organizations for assistance, information and advice. There are also childbirth education associations that can provide information for parents comtemplating another pregnancy.

To list all of these organizations here is not possible. However, parents may wish to consult guides listing these organizations; such books are available in most libraries. Two excellent guides are:

Burkas, J.L. *The Help Book.* New York: Charles Scribner's Sons, 1979.

Evans, Glen. *The Family Circle Guide to Self-Help.* New York: Ballantine Books, 1979.

* A more complete listing of resources available for premature babies and their parents may be obtained from Parents of Prematures, c/o Houston Organization for Parent Education, Inc., 3311 Richmond Avenue, Suite 330, Houston, Texas 77098.

SEWING FOR PREMIES

Clothing the premature infant is no easy task. With few exceptions, national clothing manufacturers make garments for full-term newborns. The obvious alternative is doll clothing; however most doll fashions are not acceptable attire for premies. The fabric is too stiff, the trims too scratchy, the closures inappropriate and the durability questionable.

One solution to this problem is to make the clothes. Patterns for premie clothing may be difficult to find. Some are available either free or for a slight charge from the following sources:

> Parents of Prematures
> Houston Organization for Parent Education, Inc.
> 3311 Richmond, Suite 330
> Houston, Texas 77098

> Parents of Prematures
> 13613 N.E. 26th Place
> Bellevue, Washington 98005

The pattern included in this section is among several available from Parents of Prematures, Houston.

For different styles, you may wish to make your own patterns. If you know nothing about pattern design and can find no one to create a new pattern, purchase a simple doll pattern prepared by a national pattern designer. Such patterns are sized according to the height of the doll. Choose the size which corresponds to the infant for whom garments will be made.

The following are some average measurements for a 2- to 4-pound baby. This information can be used to improvise a pattern or to give instructions to distant relatives who may want to sew for the baby.

Top of head to neck:	6″ to 6½″
Head circumference:	13″
Chest circumference:	10″
Length for shirt:	5″
Length for gown:	8″
Length of foot:	2″ to 2½″ x 1″ wide
Neckline opening:	9″

Patterns for a 15-inch or 18-inch doll need to be altered to fit a real baby.

Before beginning to sew, check with the nursery staff for any particular requirements they may have concerning clothing. Remember that the baby will be examined frequently, which requires garments that are easily opened.

FABRIC SELECTION

1. Determine whether or not to use flame retardant fabrics.
2. While baby is in an incubator, keep to fabrics cool and breathable. Nylon, rayon and 100 percent polyester are not porous and become very hot to wear. Such fabrics are better when baby is home and needs extra warmth. Cotton-and-polyester blends are fine for use in the hospital.
3. Popular color choices are pinks, greens and whites; blue tends to reflect an alarming hue onto the baby and yellow may emphasize the skin coloring of a jaundiced baby.

STYLE

1. Avoid elasticized or drawstring neck closures, and ribbons that tie at the neckline. They are hard to tie and can be dangerous.
2. Determine the position of the closure. Some staffs prefer garments that open in back while others recommend front closures. If a front closure is required and the pattern shows a back closure, sew the back pieces together along the center back line. Add a ⅝-inch seam allowance before cutting the front pattern piece in half. The seam allowance is used for the self-facing to which fasteners are attached.

FASTENERS

1. Velcro is the easiest type of fastener to use, especially while baby is in an incubator.
2. Snaps are acceptable if they do not touch baby's skin. In a heated incubator, they could burn the skin.
3. Buttons are satisfactory but take more time to close.

FINISHING

1. Garments need to be washed often so construct carefully to maintain durability.
2. Keep seams smooth so as not to irritate baby's tender skin. Protect from fraying by binding or overcasting seam edges.
3. Select soft laces or ribbons for trim. Scratchy trims near neck or arm openings can irritate skin and possibly cause a rash. Embroidery or ready-made decorations may be added for a decorative touch.

INSTRUCTIONS FOR INTENSIVE CARE GOWN

This pattern can be lengthened or shortened and garment may be worn with opening in the front if baby is hooked up to monitors.

You will need ¼ yd. or a scrap of soft, lightweight fabric . . .

2 small Velcro dots or

   small (4/0) snaps for fasteners.

Trim — as desired. Avoid scratchy lace. Bias tape is ideal.

1. Stitch shoulder seams

2. Fold under and stitch back facings in place.

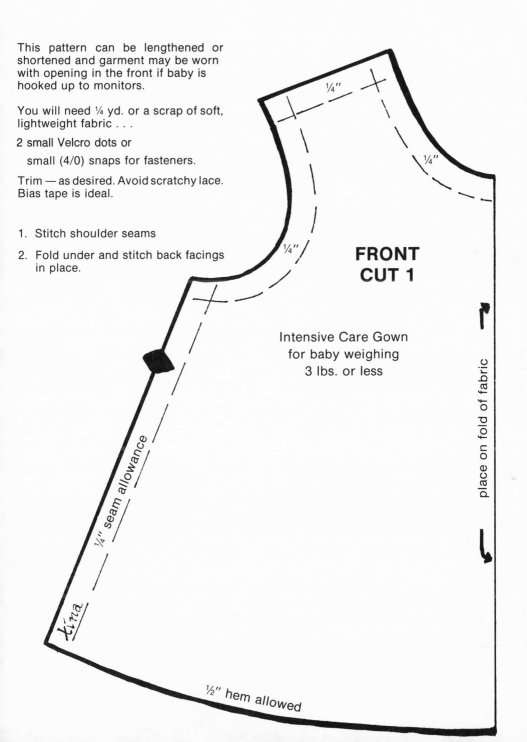

¼"

¼"

¼"

**FRONT
CUT 1**

Intensive Care Gown
for baby weighing
3 lbs. or less

place on fold of fabric

¼" seam allowance

extra

½" hem allowed

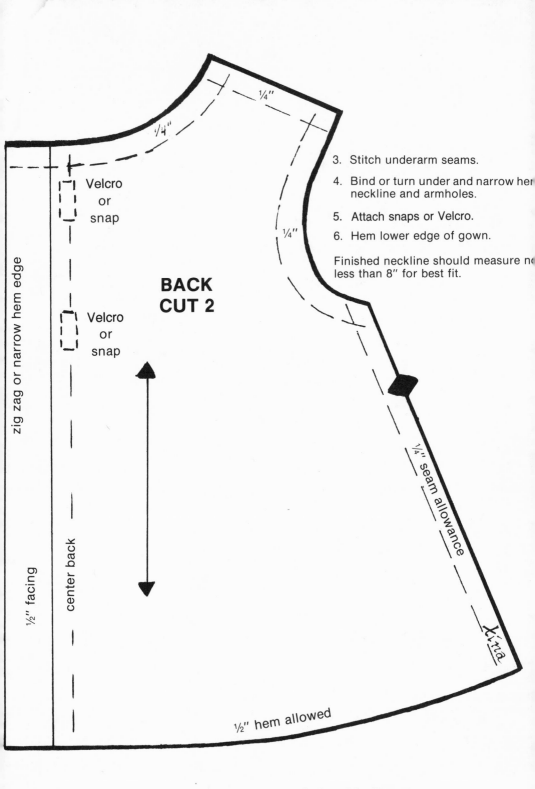

zig zag or narrow hem edge

¼"

¼"

Velcro or snap

¼"

Velcro or snap

BACK CUT 2

½" facing

center back

¼" seam allowance

Tina

½" hem allowed

3. Stitch underarm seams.

4. Bind or turn under and narrow hem neckline and armholes.

5. Attach snaps or Velcro.

6. Hem lower edge of gown.

Finished neckline should measure no less than 8" for best fit.

. . . designed by Tina Kauffman

KNITTING OR CROCHETING

When knitting or crocheting, use a newborn- or three-month-size pattern. Then use needles or hooks that are about three sizes smaller so the overall garment will come out smaller. Be careful that the neck opening does not become too small.

Once garment requirements are established and you are ready to sew, make one garment in each size. Ask the nursery staff to suggest alterations to the finished product. Adjustments may be needed for the neck openings, sleeves or overall length to accommodate a particular infant.

Providing clothing for premies can become a group sewing project for support groups and other nonprofit organizations such as Girl Scouts, Campfire Girls, church sewing circles, Red Cross volunteers and school home economics classes.

It is much more economical to make your own garments; however, you may purchase ready-made premie-size clothing from several manufacturers. See Resources, p.—— for more information.

PARENTS OF PREMATURES STATISTICAL SURVEY, MAY 1981*

In an effort to develop statistics for the community about the needs of parents of premature infants, Parents of Prematures, a service group of the Houston Organization for Parent Education, Inc., conducted a survey among families with premature children.

In 1978 and 1979 approximately 400 eight-page questionnaires were sent to parents of premature infants in Houston and to parent support groups in California, Illinois, Indiana, Iowa, Texas, Virginia and Washington.

One hundred responses were received from parents whose premature babies were born between March 1974 and August 1979. Over half of the births occurred during 1978. Twenty-seven percent of the responses received were from outside the greater Houston metropolitan area.

Of the parents who responded to this survey, most were white middle- to upper-middle-class between the ages of twenty-five and thirty-five. All respondents were ages twenty-one to fifty-one. All of the mothers received prenatal care, most beginning before eight weeks of pregnancy and continuing regularly, on at least a monthly basis.

The following is information gathered from 100 question-naires. Only definite responses to each question were tabulated. Not all parents answered all questions. Some parents gave more than one answer for some questions.

PARENT INFORMATION

Was the mother also premature?

| 2 (don't know) | 18 (yes) | 80 (no) |

Was the father also premature?

| 4 (don't know) | 7 (yes) | 89 (no) |

Is the mother a DES daughter?

| 19 (don't know) | 9 (yes) | 72 (no) |

PREGNANCY (MOTHER)

Reason delivered prematurely: (Some listed more than one cause.)

no known reason	24
membranes ruptured	19
incompetent cervix	18
multiple birth	16
toxemia	11
placenta previa	9
malformed uterus	8
abruptio placentae (separation)	7
preeclampsia	6
marginal placenta previa	4
diabetes	2
other	14

high blood pressure(2)   polyhydramnios
Bright's disease   possible kidney/bladder
infectious hepatitis   infection
hypertension   placenta may have quit
C-section done too early   functioning
repeat C-section   umbilical blood clot
possible hepatitis   intestinal infection
possible endometriosis   deep vein phlebitis
tilted uterus   ruptured abdominal abscess

Complications during pregnancy:

none	45
spotting, bleeding (excessive)	22
water leakage	14
excessive nausea	10
excessive cramping	5
severe renal problems	1
other	32

Medications taken during pregnancy:

none	4
vitamins	84
Tylenol	38
nausea medication	33
antihistamines	14
antibiotics	13
aspirin	13
other	40

Any tests done during pregnancy:

none	51*
*besides routine OB work-up	
sonography	45
amniocentesis	11
X ray	9
other	14

Did the mother smoke during pregnancy?

18 (yes)   82 (no)

Did the mother consume more than one alcoholic drink per day?

3* (yes)   97 (no)
*All specified on doctor's orders.

Was infant's movement in utero excessively active?

33 (yes)   61 (no)

When did the mother start prenatal care?

0–6 weeks	48
6–8 weeks	31
8–12 weeks	14

How often did the mother see the OB during pregnancy?

every week	3
every 2 weeks	14
every 3 weeks	13
every 4 weeks	59
every 6 weeks	1
every 8 weeks	1
other	7*

*regularly, ten times in pregnancy, three times, etc.

LABOR AND DELIVERY

Was anything done by doctor's orders to prevent or attempt to stop labor? (Some listed more than one: one mother listed seven things.)

nothing	39
bed rest	38
hospitalization	33

alcohol drip	26
alcohol by mouth	11
McDonald stitch	9
Demerol	6
Valium	5
other	9

Was the mother given hormones or shots before the baby's birth to prevent respiratory problems?

19 (yes)   81 (no)

Medications taken during labor:

none	34
not applicable	21
Demerol	19
alcohol	18
Valium	6
don't know	6
other	11

Was a fetal monitor used during labor?

11 (N/A)   5 (don't know)   70 (yes)   14 (no)

Type of delivery:

vaginal	67
C-section	33

Anesthesia for delivery: Some listed more than one, especially for delivery of twins.

none	16
epidural	23
general	23
local	16
spinal	13
gas	9
caudal	4

pudendal	3
don't know	1
other	2

Were forceps used? (Answer for each baby)

18 (N/A)   9 (don't know)   21 (yes)   56 (no)

Any complications during delivery? (Some listed more than one complication for single or twin births.)

none	54
breech	28
lack of oxygen	13
cord around neck	5
other presentations	4
other	13

Did the mother see the baby at birth?

64 (yes)   47 (no)

Did the father see the baby at birth?

53 (yes)   58 (no)

(Twins cause more than one answer in some cases.)
How long after delivery before the mother was able to see the baby?

immediately (within 1 hour)	11
1–6 hours	21
6–12 hours	11
12–24 hours	10
next day	9
3 days	19
3–7 days	11
2 weeks	1
3 weeks	1

How long after delivery before the father was able to see the baby?

immediately (within 1 hour)	72
1–6 hours	18
6–12 hours	8
12–24 hours	1

3 days	11
don't know	1

When was the first time the mother touched the baby?

immediately (within 1 hour)	15
1–6 hours	11
6–12 hours	9
12–24 hours	8
next day	17
2–3 days	18
3–7 days	15
1–2 weeks	2
2–3 weeks	2

When was the first time the mother held the baby?

immediately (within 1 hour)	7 (All specified at birth.)
1–6 hours	2
6–12 hours	4
12–24 hours	6
next day	6
2–3 days	8
3–7 days	17
1–2 weeks	8
2–4 weeks	10
4–8 weeks	9
over 2 months	3
not yet	1
after death	1

Was the baby transferred to another hospital?

52 (yes)   53 (no)

Who was the parent's first contact for information concerning the baby's status?

doctor	87
nurse	9
don't know	1
ICU	1
Parents of Prematures	1
husband	1

BABY INFORMATION

There were a total of 100 sets of parents. Two families gave statistics for two separate births each so responses include 102 births.

number of babies in survey	119
female	54
male	63
sex not stated	2
single births	86
sets of twins	15
sets of triplets	1
deaths	11*

*two after several months, one from SIDS

CONVERSION OF POUNDS AND OUNCES TO GRAMS

		pounds						
		0	1	2	3	4	5	6
	0	—	454	907	1361	1814	2268	2722
	1	28	482	936	1389	1843	2296	2750
	2	57	510	964	1417	1871	2325	2778
	3	85	539	992	1446	1899	2353	2807
	4	113	567	1021	1474	1928	2381	2835
	5	142	595	1049	1503	1956	2410	2863
Ounces	6	170	624	1077	1531	1984	2438	2892
	7	198	652	1106	1559	2013	2466	2920
	8	227	680	1134	1588	2041	2495	2948
	9	255	709	1162	1616	2070	2523	2977
	10	283	737	1191	1644	2098	2551	3005
	11	312	765	1219	1673	2126	2580	3033

CONVERSION OF POUNDS AND OUNCES TO GRAMS (CON'T)

	pounds						
	0	1	2	3	4	5	6
12	340	794	1247	1701	2155	2608	3062
13	369	822	1276	1729	2183	2637	3090
14	397	850	1304	1758	2211	2665	3118
15	425	879	1332	1786	2240	2693	3147

BIRTH WEIGHTS

weight in pounds and ounces	number of babies
1-9 to 1-15	10
2-0 to 2-7	16
2-8 to 2-15	24
3-0 to 3-7	17
3-8 to 3-15	11
4-0 to 4-7	14
4-8 to 4-15	14
5-0 to 5-7	3
5-8 to 5-15	3
6-0 to 8-1	4

GOING-HOME WEIGHT

weight in pounds and ounces	number of babies
3-7 (lowest)	2
3-8 to 3-15	11
4-0 to 4-7	30
4-8 to 4-15	33
5-0 to 5-7	18
5-8 to 5-15	3
6-0 to 6-7	1
6-8 to 6-15	1
7-0 to 7-7	6
9-0	1

WEEKS EARLY

number of weeks	number of babies
2	1
3	3
4	7
5	6
6	5
7	10
8	21
9	7
10	11
11	15
12	7
13	3
14	2
15	2
16	1
17	1

HOW LONG IN HOSPITAL

number of weeks	number of babies
1 or less	7
1–2	15
2–3	8
3–4	8
4–6	20
6–8	20
8–12	21
12–16	4
16–18	2
Still at time of survey	4

Baby's problems following birth:

none	1
body temperature	81
jaundice	63
respiratory distress	62
apnea	58
immature lungs	49
slow weight gain	47
no sucking, rooting reflex	45
hyaline membrane disease	45
anemia	39

bradycardia episodes	37
heart murmur	30
open ductus	19
required exchange transfusion	17*
*one baby had nine transfusions	
IVH	12
pneumothorax	7**
**one baby had five episodes—counted as one	
hydrocephalus	5
physical abnormality	4
other (some listed several)	22

bronchopulmonary dysplasia (4)
interstitial emphysema (3)
hernia (2)
retinopathy of prematurity (2)
IRDS (2)
seizures (2)
small trachea
blood disorder
gas-caused rapid heartbeat
spitting up milk
hypertension
hyperthyroid
group B strep infection
dextrocardia
bladder infection
severe diarrhea
no white blood cells for weeks
liver biopsy
severe eye infection

meningitis
bowel adhesion (minor)
inability to thrive
developmental delay
skin disease (systematic
epidural neures)
pneumonia
brain damage
surgery
NEC
acidosis
too much blood
hypoglycemia
sepsis
pseudomonius infection
abnormal distension
required oxygen
TE fistula

Was this the mother's firstborn?

58 (yes)   42 (no)

OTHER CHILDREN

Number of mothers who had previously

given birth	42
had a premature baby	13

had a miscarriage   27
had a stillbirth   5

PUMPING

Did the mother pump breast milk?

68 (yes)   34 (no)

Was the mother given a dry-up shot after delivery?

25 (yes)   75 (no)

What pump was used? (Some listed more than one.)

not applicable   23
electric   41
rubber bulb (suction)   36
Loyd-B   28
other   4
hand expression (1)

Was the pump used satisfactory?

58 (yes)   16 (no)

Did the mother have adequate pumping information?

58 (yes)   17 (no)

Who provided pumping information?

La Leche League   26
hospital   15
nurse   9
POP member   7
pump distributor   3
pump instructions   3
doctor   2
HOPE   2
book or manual   1
friend   1
breast consultant   1
previous experience   1

Would the mother have preferred a different pump?

19 (yes)   47 (no)

Was the mother successful at pumping?

38 (yes)   4 (no)   27 (somewhat)

After delivery, was the mother encouraged to pump?

60 (yes)   30 (no)

How long after delivery did pumping begin?

within 24 hours	34
2–3 days	26
more than 3 days	9

How often did the mother pump?

every 2–3 hours	32
every 4–5 hours	32
less than 5 times daily	8

How long did the mother pump each time?

less than 10 minutes	10
10–20 minutes	38
25–40 minutes	22
45–75 minutes	2

Breast-Pumping Tips Offered by Survey Respondents

Most of the mothers who responded to this question had the following advice (listed in order of most common responses):

Don't get discouraged; keep working at it. The whole process can be very frustrating, but it is worth it.

Get plenty of rest.

Relax.

Drink plenty of fluids.

Get adequate information. Ask for help if necessary.

Get a good pump; if one doesn't work effectively, try another.

Start early and pump regularly.

Talk to others who have been through it for additional support.

Use various methods to find what works best—try hot showers or baths for relaxation, deep hot massage of breasts to prevent or relieve engorgement. Look at a photo of your baby while pumping. Use nipple stimulation. Massage breasts while pumping.

Remember, you can change your mind. If the process is too stressful, at least you have tried; and it may be in your own best interest to stop.

NURSING

After delivery, was the mother encouraged to nurse?

44 (yes)   50 (no)

Did the mother plan to nurse before the premature birth?

58 (yes)   26 (no)   12 (undecided)

How long after delivery before the mother was allowed to nurse?

didn't nurse	36
unable to nurse	11
within one week	14
2–4 weeks	19
5–8 weeks	11
9–12 weeks	5

Did the mother successfully nurse?

36 (yes)   23 (no)   2 (somewhat)

(Of those who answered this question, one mother of twins said yes for one baby and no for the other. A mother who nursed for three months considered herself unsuccessful while another who nursed for two weeks felt successful at nursing.)

How long did the mother nurse?

still nursing	15
1–6 weeks	9
2–5 months	11
6–12 months	5
other	7*

*answers up to eighteen months

Did the mother nurse and supplement?

38 (yes)   17 (no)

Some of the reasons given for supplementing:

inverted nipples
lack of milk
easier to feed with bottle
breast-milk jaundice
baby not getting enough breast milk
alternating twins
breast milk in bottle given for a while

Nineteen mothers had successfully nursed a previous baby. Nursing tips offered by survey respondents (listed in order of most common response first):

Most mothers felt one thing to be most important in breast feeding a premie: patience.

It can take much time and patience to get a premie to nurse.

Take time and be calm. Don't force the baby.

Get help, advice, support from others who have done it.

Keep trying. Get rest and drink fluids.

Try different nursing positions.

"Let down" milk before putting baby to the breast.

Massage breasts gently while nursing to increase milk flow.

Use nursing for baby's "comfort" too, once established.

Don't get frustrated about supplementing—milk is most important; the method is secondary. You can give baby bottles with breast milk you have pumped.

Take time to appreciate your baby and realize the ultimate benefit of breast-feeding.

FOLLOW-UP

Baby's development so far:

normal	83
slow	20
advanced	1
died	2

Problems:

none	22
colic	41
ear infections	26
constipation	21
required surgery	19

ear tubes	gastrostomy
hernia	retina
ductus closed	eyes and ears
other heart surgery	TE fistula
plastic	shunt
imperforated anus	for NEC

eye problems	15
respiratory infections	15
required therapy	15

physical (some for   infant stimulation
cerebral palsy)   inhalation
speech   phototherapy (later)

frequent illness	11
excessive temper tantrums	10
muscular weaknesses	9
diarrhea (chronic)	7
seizures	7
heart problems	5
hearing	4
hyperactivity	4
speech	4
other	28

episodes of pallor   swallowing
little sleep   stitches surfacing
very active (not hyper)   lactose intolerance
hospitalized again   late talker
small facial lump   slow motor development
developmental center   slow growth, size
 program   apnea—required monitor
allergies   and therapy at home
chronic spitting up   wheezing
postural drainage   asthma
shunt obstructions   whooping cough
acidosis   excess tone on one side
difficulty coordinating   congestion

Any problems directly related to prematurity or birth trauma:

none	77
hydrocephalus	6
lungs	6
eye problems	4
(retina burns, blindness, etc.)	
cerebral palsy	4
retardation	1
other	6

Age at which baby was first taken out in public:

not yet	2
1–4 weeks	16
5–8 weeks	19
9–12 weeks	27
longer	33

Approximately what was the total bill from the hospital only?

Answers ranged from $150 to $250,000.

Most were between $5,000 and $30,000.

Other

During your child's first year after birth, what have been your problems of most concern?

The overwhelming concern was of specific illnesses— ear infections, frequent colds, respiratory infections, eye problems, colic, allergies, etc.

A close second concern was of development and growth. (One mother said "to allow him to develop at his own speed in his own direction. Not overfeed, over-protect or underdiscipline.") Three parents expressed concern about retardation.

A third concern was whether there would be future problems resulting from prematurity.

Other concerns less commonly expressed were about diet, sleep, daily routine problems, discipline, worry about having another child, concern for a child who is still terrified of doctors and hospitals, isolation during the first year, fear of possible infections, going out in public, parental fatigue, difficulty getting baby-sitters, bonding, fear of not caring for the baby properly, and finances.

Any comments, concerns, suggestions, feelings:
There were sixty different responses to this question. The most common subject was that of the benefits of a parent support group, either

saying how much it helped, how much it would have helped if the parents had known to contact such a group at the time they needed it, or suggesting that parents seek support from other parents who have been through a similar experience.

The next most common type of response was telling what the parents had experienced themselves and giving suggestions for how to cope. These responses varied from tales of actual illnesses of the mother and babies to how the parents dealt with friends, relatives and professionals to observations on the baby's development during the first year or so. Parents admonished against comparisons of the premie with any other children, while encouraging medical evaluation of and seeking help for the baby whose development is slow.

Other concerns mentioned include matters of health, discipline, responsibility, finances and a fear of future problems related to prematurity.

There were several suggestions about the need for more written material about prematurity and how parents can cope, for more statistical information, for parents' need for education concerning the baby's problems and what to expect, and the need for before/after bulletin boards in the hospital for baby photos.

To obtain copies of the original "Parent Information File" questionnaire used for this survey or additional copies of the survey results, write to:

> Parents of Prematures
> c/o HOPE
> 3311 Richmond, Suite 330
> Houston, Texas 77098
> Enclose $ for each copy to cover printing and mailing costs.

*© 1981 by Joanne Williams, Susan Kahn and Tina Kauffman. Used by permission.

INDEX